Dior

PERFUME

To my mother, who only ever wore Miss Dior.

Slipcase front: Detail of an advertisement for Miss Dior perfume, illustrated by René Gruau. Photo © SARL René Gruau/www.renegruau.com.
Slipcase back: *Dovima with elephants, evening dress by Dior, Cirque d'Hiver, Paris, August 1955*. Photo © The Richard Avedon Foundation.
Following pages: The first Christian Dior amphora perfume bottle, 1947. Photo © Laziz Hamani.
© 2012 Assouline Publishing
601 West 26th Street, 18th floor
New York, NY 10001, USA
Tel.: 212-989-6810 Fax: 212-647-0005
www.assouline.com
Color separation by Luc Alexis Chasleries.
Text translated from the French by Gail de Courcy-Ireland.
Captions written by Vincent Leret.
Printed in China.
ISBN: 9781614280286
All rights reserved. No part of this publication may be reproduced or transmitted in any form or by any means, electronic or otherwise, without prior consent of the publisher.

Jérôme Hanover

Dior

PERFUME

ASSOULINE

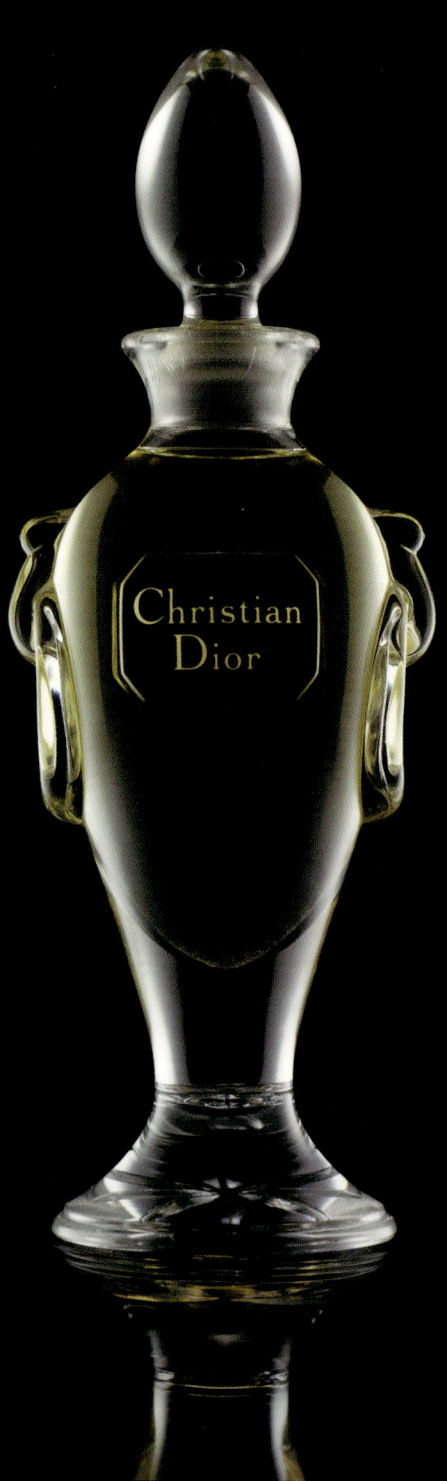

> *All of Dior's perfumes uphold their initial legacy: to be very couture, very Dior.*

a thick white mantle cloaks the setting; Avenue Montaigne seems to want to match the sable coats of the elegant ladies hurrying down it. Paris is covered in snow. Just one week ago, temperatures dropped to 7° Fahrenheit. At number 30, the atmosphere is heady with excitement: In a matter of days, Christian Dior will present his first haute couture show, and his team is busy making sure it will be as perfect as Monsieur wants it. "Will he make his mark?" is the question no doubt running through everybody's minds, from the seamstress stitching earnestly away, to the couturier, stressed by the stakes at play. We now know that February 12, 1947, would go down in history, but at the time uncertainty reigned. Christian Dior had a new vision of women: not simply of the female figure, but of a woman's presence overall. Haute couture would dress her, while perfume would accompany her, lingering in her wake. Sometimes it would even precede her: In his new store, where the final adjustments were being made for the upcoming opening, a full liter of perfume would be sprayed every week—the very fragrance that would cast its spell over Dior's salons during the couture event of the year, which posterity has recorded as the New Look. Perfume would complement Dior's vision of style, it would be its prolongation in scent—more still, its match. Christian Dior took such care and time over this fragrance, no one could underrate its significance in relation to fashion. The two would progress side by side, in mutual enrichment and inspiration. In the pearl-gray salons on the third floor, Christian Dior's mind was racing. With the last fittings came the final tweaks to the dresses. Small questions could not turn into big issues, yet still there was no name for this perfume, a floral green chypre. Within a few dozen hours, this new fragrance would be to perfumery what the first Dior couture show became to fashion, but the reason it was still being referred to by its code name was not for discretion's sake. A thousand words jostled in Christian Dior's head, already adding to the overexertion that would strike him down ten years later. Which to choose? Mitzah Bricard was pacing up and down. She was his muse, his advisor, his paragon of elegance, the caryatid he could count on for support. Catching Christian's eye in the mirror above the grand marble chimneypiece, she paused to check her profile, queenly as Nefertiti. She was wearing her ubiquitous leopard-print scarf, knotted around her wrist like a *tabaquero* singing *Carmen*, a touch of brazen irony in contrast with her elegant natural allure, as if to snub the diamonds and pearls nestled beneath her blouse. The door opened a crack, quiet and discreet, typical of Catherine Dior, as she slipped in to see her brother on some long-forgotten pretext. Christian snapped out of his musing and smiled; all stress seemed to subside. He was her "Tian" and she his darling "chérie." Mademoiselle Dior. Twelve years his junior. Mitzah Bricard, whose mother was English, rose from her Médaillon chair: "Ah, here's Miss Dior!" she exclaimed. Miss Dior? Miss Dior! All was ready: The show could go on. "Outfit number one…"

> Christian Dior's legacy to the house he founded is a creative universe, a vision of perfumery intimately linked to his fashion.

Miss Dior is a perfume manifesto, but not simply because it was the House of Dior's first fragrance. It clearly states the couturier's intention to turn perfumery into a fashion accessory, an indispensable item of luxury. Since its creation, over seventy other fragrances or variations have been born.

From eaux de toilette to absolutes, colognes to extracts, all of Dior's perfumes uphold their initial legacy: to be very couture, very Dior.

"Perfume is the indispensable complement to the personality of women, the finishing touch on a dress."[1] In Christian Dior's wildest dreams, he would have been able to create a fragrance for each of the looks in his couture show. This couldn't happen, of course, for fashion and perfumery play on very different time scales.[2] Yet the ultimate fantasy has been transposed within the House of Dior through a very clear bond between the two departments. Yards of exceptional materials for one, a rigorous selection of the most precious ingredients for the other.[3] In the postwar years when going without—be it clothes or perfumes—was still an everyday reality for French ladies, Christian Dior reinvented luxury and dreams. This new statement required a new language. His perfume was like his vision of fashion: iconoclastic, imposing accords and constructions that often flouted the prevailing perfumery canons. Yet just as his New Look broke with the fashion of the day to draw inspiration from the dresses of the Belle Époque, his fragrances traveled back in time to fully translate the influence of perfume history into a modern olfactory language. So it was for Diorissimo. When it arrived on the pearl-gray shelves of Dior boutiques in 1956, this perfume composed by Edmond Roudnitska both inspired and enthralled. Youngsters loved the fragrance: It was like nothing they had ever known. "I worked with fresh, light notes, clear and flowing, purely olfactory, and avoiding any heavy, gustative effects," explained the perfume's creator. "I monitored each link between the different accords to bring out a kind of olfactory melody and ensure an overall unity to the perfume's form."[4] Diorissimo goes straight to the heart; it is a clean, absolute floral. "It opens with fresh green notes of soil and crumpled leaves that hook you in. A clear, clean *sillage* takes over. The theme is an armful of lily of the valley. It intoxicates, plays on jasmine, orange blossom, rose, and lilac, becoming heady and more intense, heavier and more sensual, deeper and more animal. There is a form of olfactory expression, signature, and style that shines forth beyond the theme. The components are mastered and contain a perfect sequence, a deep olfactory knowledge of a sprig of lily of the valley, picked at dawn and inhaled until the evening."[5] As a perfume narrative that spins the story of a day in the flower's life, Diorissimo instantly put all the heavy, grandiloquent constructions of its peers out of fashion: It is a romantic fragrance with a tight, coherent vocabulary, a perfume that could have been made in the nineteenth century. At the time, the absence of gustative notes (vanilla, sweet, or fruity) stood out against most contemporary creations because its pedigree traveled even further back in time, to the days before synthetic molecules.[6] "I decided to break with most of the products that had been overused," concluded Edmond Roudnitska about Diorissimo.[7] Didn't Christian Dior have the very same thing in mind when revolutionizing and redefining the female figure in each of his couture shows?

From then on, the visual identity had to be the same for both worlds. While this approach can today seem self-evident in a fragrance market heavily influenced by fashion labels, which see perfumes as an extension of their textile proposal, back in the postwar years, when the first Dior perfumes were born, it was far from obvious. Christian Dior was not the first couturier to feel he was a perfumer: Nina Ricci, Pierre Balmain, Cristobal Balenciaga, Gabrielle Chanel, and others had created perfumes, and Elsa Schiaparelli even chose names for each of her fragrances that started with her own initial (Shocking, Snuff, Souci, Salut...) and stamped her signature pink throughout. But for most of the above, the only thing that was couture about a perfume was its luxuriousness and its name. Christian Dior thought otherwise. Although his fragrances were an olfactory translation of his fashion world, for most women this correlation was rather esoteric. To know it, you had to see it. Posed majestically on pleated gray silk, the womanly curves of the original Miss Dior bottle, designed by Fernand Guéry-Colas in 1947, seem to highlight a hipline magnified by the basque of a Bar suit. In 1950, a new design asserted the influence from fashion even more distinctly: The geometrically structured, square-shaped bottle was inspired by the Vertical line.[8] Its frosted glass reproduces the houndstooth motif favored by Christian Dior, an originally masculine check to which he brought feminine grace and sensuality. A pretty couture bow adorns the bottle neck: All the House of Dior codes are there, as though the perfume itself is dressed in Dior. Taking the analogy of perfumes as dresses further, Christian Dior blended them into the world of couture by having their bottles echo the atmosphere and details in the salons at 30 Avenue Montaigne, like a string of mini-boutiques. The dominant Trianon gray and white, the medallion inspired by the backs of the neo–Louis XVI chairs... The black and white packaging of Eau Fraîche may seem a far cry from the *cannage*, or cane-work, on the concert-hall chairs in Dior Haute Couture shows, yet it adopts the rattan furniture motif of which the couturier was so fond. The exact Napoleon III weave motif has been honored on the different Escales bottles since 2008.⁹ And when the people at Dior imagined a new version of Miss Dior Chérie in 2011, they made the couture identity clearly apparent, all the way down to the stylized embroidery on the perfume's posters and packaging.

> " A pretty couture bow adorns the bottle neck: All the House of Dior codes are there, as though the perfume itself is dressed in Dior. "

"Naturally, the dress can correspond to the name it bears… but these christenings have not always been purposefully thought out," Christian Dior explained. "The dresses start out with a number; we don't name them until they start to come to life, in order to differentiate them the further they are in the making."¹⁰ Indeed, the name the couturier gave should not be interpreted as a literal description. More than one dress or outfit has been named Rosée, meaning "dew" in

French, which seems to evoke the fresh morning dewdrops in a garden—yet they have all been evening wear. We could argue that the lady may have danced the night away in her organdy dress stitched with *broderie anglaise*, only returning home at dawn, or that Christian Dior was perhaps playing on the irony in this paradox.[11] We could even imagine the drops of dew that appear on plants and flowers in the first flush of day, as though having drunk their scent all night long: Is this not the perfect metaphor for perfume? But fun as it may be to hypothesize on the interpretation of this or that name the couturier father gave his fashion offspring, it is the recurring vocabulary from the Dior lexicon, collection after collection, which tells us most about Christian Dior's intentions. In the decade from 1947 to 1957, over three hundred couture outfits bore a name linked to perfumery, with flowers uppermost among them—the flowers that compose the house fragrances. The gardenia and patchouli found in Miss Dior are also a day suit and an afternoon dress respectively.[12] The mandarin in Eau Fraîche gave its name, Mandarine, to a chiffon outfit and a black woolen coat.[13] The lily of the valley in Diorissimo, Muguet, has been a lingerie gown, a fur *paletot*, two evening gowns, and a short-skirted outfit.[14] There have been Acacia, Marguerite, Pétunia, Réséda, Myosotis, Lys, Iris, Coquelicot, Dahlia, Hortensia, Lupin, Œillet, Colza, Bouton d'or, Angélique, Scabieuse,[15] and an endless array of roses: Roseraie, Rosée, Rose de France, Damascus Rose, Christmas Rose, April or Brabant Rose, Tea Rose, Black Rose or Red Rose, Rose Pompon, Nuit Rose, Fête des Roses, Soirée Rose, Palais Rose, La Vie en Rose, and even Fontenay-aux-Roses—a southern suburb of Paris! Virtually every scented flower that exists seems to have lent its name to at least one Dior dress. In the elite haute couture that all women dream of but only few can wear, city flowers mix with country blooms: Sported prettily in a buttonhole, found in the wild during a stroll, planted in endless lush flowerbeds, simple or sophisticated; every flower is beautiful, Christian Dior seems to say, every flower smells lovely. To echo the names of these outfits that recall perfumery's soliflores—fragrances created around a single flower—he created his own bouquets and evocative compositions: his very own accords. Hence Jardin Japonais, or Japanese garden, which makes it so easy to imagine the scent of blossoming cherry trees, orchids, and lotus flowers behind this afternoon dress and coat.[16] And can't you just sense the winding ivy and fresh hollyhock in this wool suit and organza blouse named Charmille, the French for "arbor"?[17] In Herbier, a beige crepe dress with matching wool suit, whose name evokes the herbariums of old, can't you snatch the scent of crisp dried flowers pressed against yellowing paper? Not to mention the Jardin de Curé, literally "priest's garden" in French, which has been at once a black alpaca coat, an evening gown, and a dinner dress?[18] Does it not echo the famous Jardin de Mon Curé, created by Jacques Guerlain in 1895, and its accords of lemon, jasmine, and ylang-ylang? Dior even adorned his dresses with the names of his own perfumes, and vice versa: Miss Dior became a cocktail dress in black faille and an evening gown embroidered with a thousand flowers, while Diorama was a black wool dress trimmed with skunk before becoming Edmond Roudnitska's first perfume for Dior.[19] The name is sported by two other dresses too: one a surat cotton dinner dress and the other featuring a black horsehair trim against a pink background.[20] The connections have persisted well beyond the couturier's death: Jules, the name of a suit in 1956, became a masculine fragrance twenty-four years later. And Chérie, which was both a suit and a dress during Christian Dior's lifetime, became the new version of Miss Dior in 2005.[21]

Christian Dior loved playing with words, starting with his own name. Soft, rounded, sensual, and glamorous, it trips off the tongue, lingers on the diphthong, then melts into the final syllable. Dior is such a euphonic name, and Christian gave his surname to all his perfumes, as though claiming their paternity. First Miss Dior, in 1947, in reference to his sister Catherine, as we have seen. Then Diorama in 1949, which now seems so closely linked to the perfume we forget that the word was first imagined by Louis Daguerre in 1822 as the name for one of his inventions, the ancestor of film, whose special way of lighting translucent panels gave the illusion of motion to the scenes portrayed, and which comes from the Greek *dia*, meaning through, and *orama*, meaning sight. It is a couture perfume for the silver screen. In 1956, Diorissimo echoed the musical annotations pianissimo (very soft) or fortissimo (very loud). In Italian, the *–issimo* suffix is the superlative, so Diorissimo should be seen as pure Dior: Dior to the power of Dior! In fact, this was probably Christian Dior's most personal perfume, featuring lily of the valley, his favorite flower, which he made sure was sewn into the lining of his dresses to bring him luck in his couture shows. His involvement even stretched to designing the spectacular bottle and its stopper, which blooms like a great bouquet of gilded flowers. Yet this perfume was also his last. By 1963, both Christian Dior and Serge Heftler-Louiche, his childhood friend and cofounder of Parfums Christian Dior, had passed away, but the spirit lived on. A new fragrance was created by Paul Vacher, the nose behind Miss Dior, still playing on the master's name once more: Diorling rings like darling. Then came Diorella, as fresh and spicy as a young woman sparkling in couture; Dior-Dior, a double-barreled Dior; and Dioressence, the utmost essence of Dior, consummate femininity. In J'adore too, no doubt, there is still a play on the name, in *adioration* of the master.

eau Sauvage was the first masculine fragrance created by Dior. The first actually made for men, many of whom—including Christian Dior himself—had already adopted Eau Fraîche, a simple, natural cologne created by Edmond Roudnitska for Dior in 1955, whose advertising and packaging played on an ambiguity between his and hers and seemed to address both. Ladies saw it as a light and sporty summer fragrance, gentlemen as a subtle, invigorating *jus* that had shed the scent of lavender, at last! Eau Fraîche had become a unisex fragrance, no doubt the first to exist on such a scale, but it had been imagined as a women's eau de toilette: a light, citrus chypre that fit the tastes of American ladies in the 1950s. When Edmond Roudnitska created Eau Sauvage thirteen tears later, he wanted to take the perfumery theory he had elaborated in creating Diorissimo—clean rigor and more olfactory notes than gustative—and apply it to men. "The characteristic of Eau Sauvage is that it is discreet and effacing but present for a very long time, floating like a gentle veil behind the person wearing it."[22] Lemon, jasmine, and vetiver: The composition was simple and strict but revolutionary. Like Eau Fraîche, Eau Sauvage is a chypre—fittingly enough, this time the ladies started borrowing the perfume from their men, arguing that the gadroon on the bottle looked like the pleats of a couture dress and the cap seemed inspired by a thimble! In 2004, Bois d'Argent, created by Annick Ménardo, and Cologne Blanche and Eau Noire, both created by Francis Kurkdjian, all had the same effect: three fragrances from the Dior Homme fashion universe that appealed to women too.

"When you're looking for a name for a perfume that can appeal to an international audience, you always come up against oppositions: All the dictionaries in the world have been copyrighted, but this name wasn't. There must be a reason. Because no one dared to take it!"[23] Poison is ripe with subversion. Controlled arrogance. The traditional gray and white associated with Dior perfumes found itself replaced by amethyst and emerald green. Poison was the first ladies' perfume that did not echo the couturier's surname. Only the medallion inspired by the backs of the neo–Louis XVI chairs in the Avenue Montaigne flagship remains on the packaging, creating a unity with the other house fragrances—like a special beauty spot that the women in a given family all have in exactly the same place. I am a Dior perfume, it clearly states. But in this new context it is perceived differently, as an oval mirror in which we imagine a wicked queen inquiring: Who is the fairest of them all? Could it be someone else? The plump, round bottle suggests the form of an apple: the poison-ed fruit. Unlike Miss Dior, Poison started life as a name, around which the fragrance and the packaging were built. A daring perfume with a potent liturgy orchestrated to provoke temptation, the fragrance had high expectations to

> "Poison started life as a name, around which the fragrance and the packaging were built. A daring perfume with a potent liturgy orchestrated to provoke temptation."

live up to: More than eight hundred proposals were made.[24] Poison wasn't going to whisper sweet nothings. Poison had to be risqué, a musky animal scent to set the pulse dizzily racing. But before reaching this sensual, bewitching end note, Poison glitters, flitters between coriander, pepper, and cinnamon accords. It weaves a mysterious web of spicy to fruity notes that create a tenacious sillage—ordinarily an oxymoron, the first evoking the persistence of the fragrance and the latter its diffuse presence. For there was never any question of Poison leaving darkness in its wake; the perfume is complex, enigmatic. It spurs an impulse for love and death in one breath. It celebrates a dangerous beauty, absolute femininity, the fantasy of Lucrezia Borgia assuaged, the Marquise de Brinvilliers brought to heel. "So what is Poison? It is nonconformism, flying in the face of convention; what we are recreating here is the Dior saga itself."[25]

Crystal chandeliers and halls of mirrors: After top model Carmen Kass's mythical bath of gold and Charlize Theron's striptease—"Gold is cold," she proclaimed at the time—the splendor of the Château de Versailles provided the setting for the latest J'adore opus in 2011. A pure concentrate of Dior aesthetics, this ninety-second film can be seen to encapsulate the saga of Dior perfumes. It clearly reaffirms the couturier's desire to associate his perfumes to his fashions: The setting is an Haute Couture runway show, reminiscent of the famous opening in 1947, when Miss Dior and the New Look redefined the canons of femininity. Close-up on Charlize Theron's towering heels as she runs through the

> *Diorling rings like darling. Then came Diorella, as fresh and spicy as a young woman sparkling in couture; Dior-Dior, a double-barreled Dior; and Dioressence, the utmost essence of Dior, consummate femininity. In J'adore too, no doubt, there is still a play on the name, in adioration of the master.*

Hall of Mirrors, sexy as hell in a chic black suit. She could be Belphegor, but really she is Diorella. Backstage, she meets the other models preparing for the show, greets Grace Kelly with a kiss, shares a look with Marlene Dietrich and Marilyn Monroe. These three actresses all wore Dior, but the marvels of technology enabled director Jean-Jacques Annaud to dress them in some of the couture house's very latest creations. Past and present tell the same story. Like this film, J'adore is quintessentially Dior. Calice Becker had only just turned thirty when she created this perfume. It is a youthful fragrance, as each of Dior's creations were likewise in their day. Bright as raw gold bullion, yet as meticulously crafted as a precious jewel. "Instead of creating a classic floral accord, I 'painted' each flower individually then brought them all together in a bouquet, to which I added a basket of lush fruit." Rose and lily of the valley are present, of course, but Christian Dior's two totemic blooms blend into a harmonious composition balanced between magnolia, violet, orchid, and carnation, a simple echo of the past. Christian Dior would have adored J'adore. He would have been transported back to his garden in Milly-la-Forêt from the very first note, an ode to his personal aesthetic and his obsession for novelty. A very twenty-first-century Dior.

Since that icy day back in February 1947, the saga of Dior perfumes reads like a great novel. Catherine, Christian's darling sister, the symbolic Miss and muse behind the limelight, kept her maiden name all life long, as though to ever remain the Miss Dior who inspired that first perfume. Christian died in 1957. Miss Dior, Diorama, Eau Fraîche, Diorissimo: Ten years brought only four fragrances, but each with its own radical approach. The result is an olfactory melody and a crystal-clear aesthetic. Christian Dior's legacy to the house he founded is a creative universe, a vision of perfumery intimately linked to his fashion. His successors have written new chapters in the story, drawing on his life and work for inspiration. Today François Demachy upholds the tradition as the house perfumer for Dior—a rare luxury. It is he who rewrites the main chapters in the House of Dior's history and dreams up those yet to come.

> In Christian Dior's wildest dreams, he would have been able to create a fragrance for each of the looks in his couture show.

"The thing I remember most about the women in my childhood is their perfumes. They had a lasting fragrance, much more so than today, filling the air in the elevator long after the ladies had stepped out."[26] This confession from the couturier leaves no doubt as to his intentions as a perfumer. Christian Dior cloaked his memories in fragrance to bring the ladies from his childhood back to life. To materialize his olfactory memory.

> **I see myself as a perfumer as much as a couturier.**
>
> Christian Dior

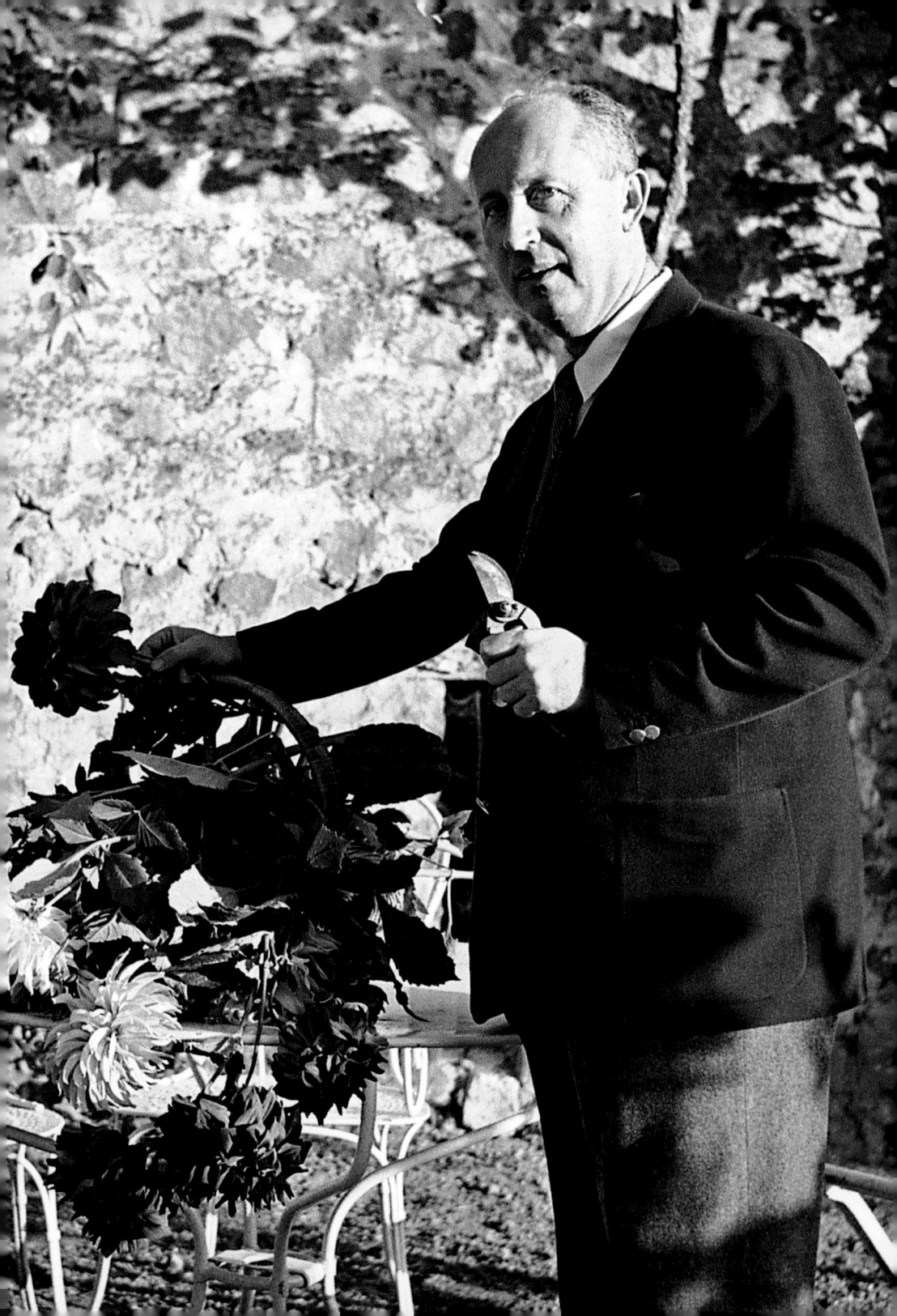

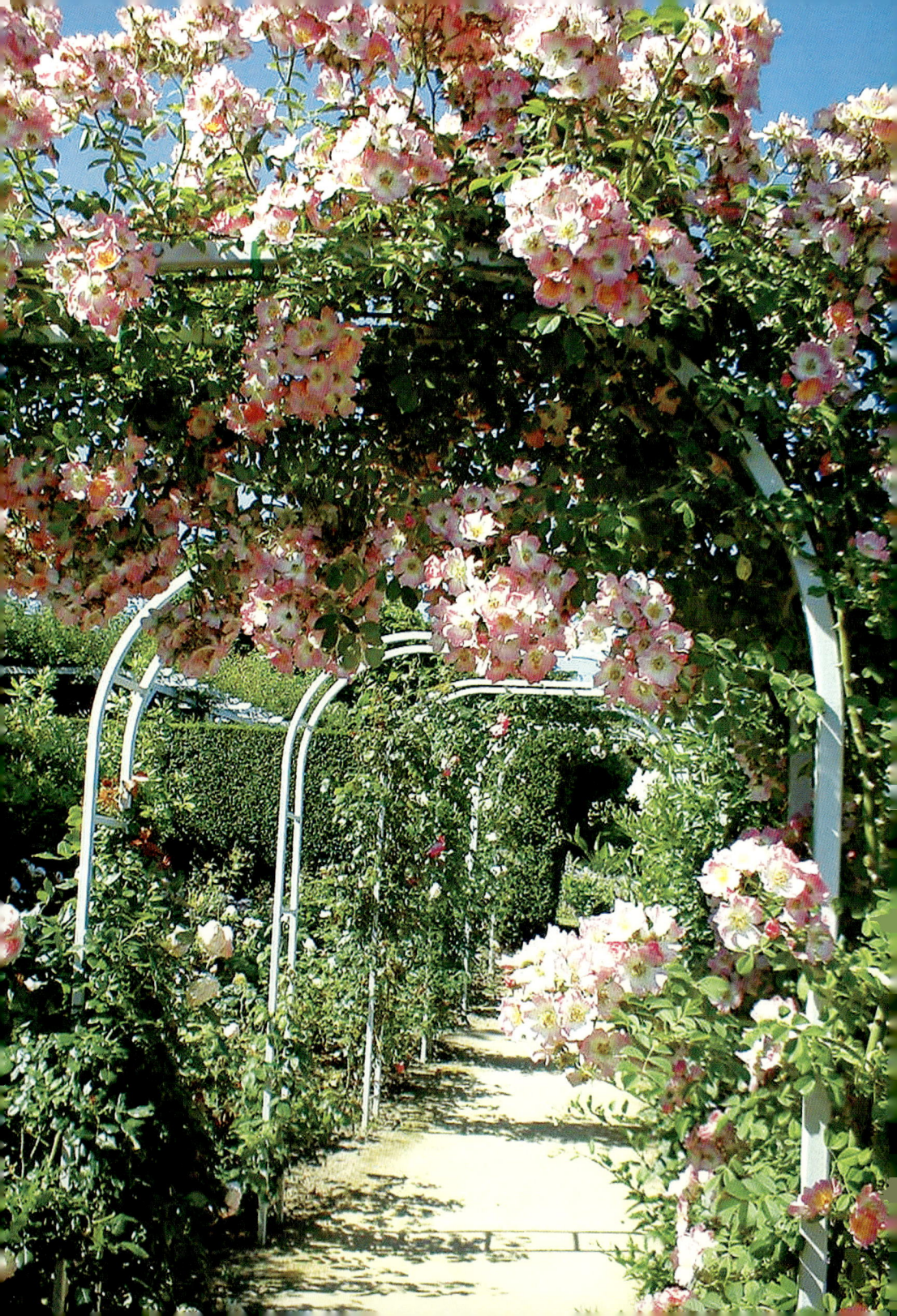

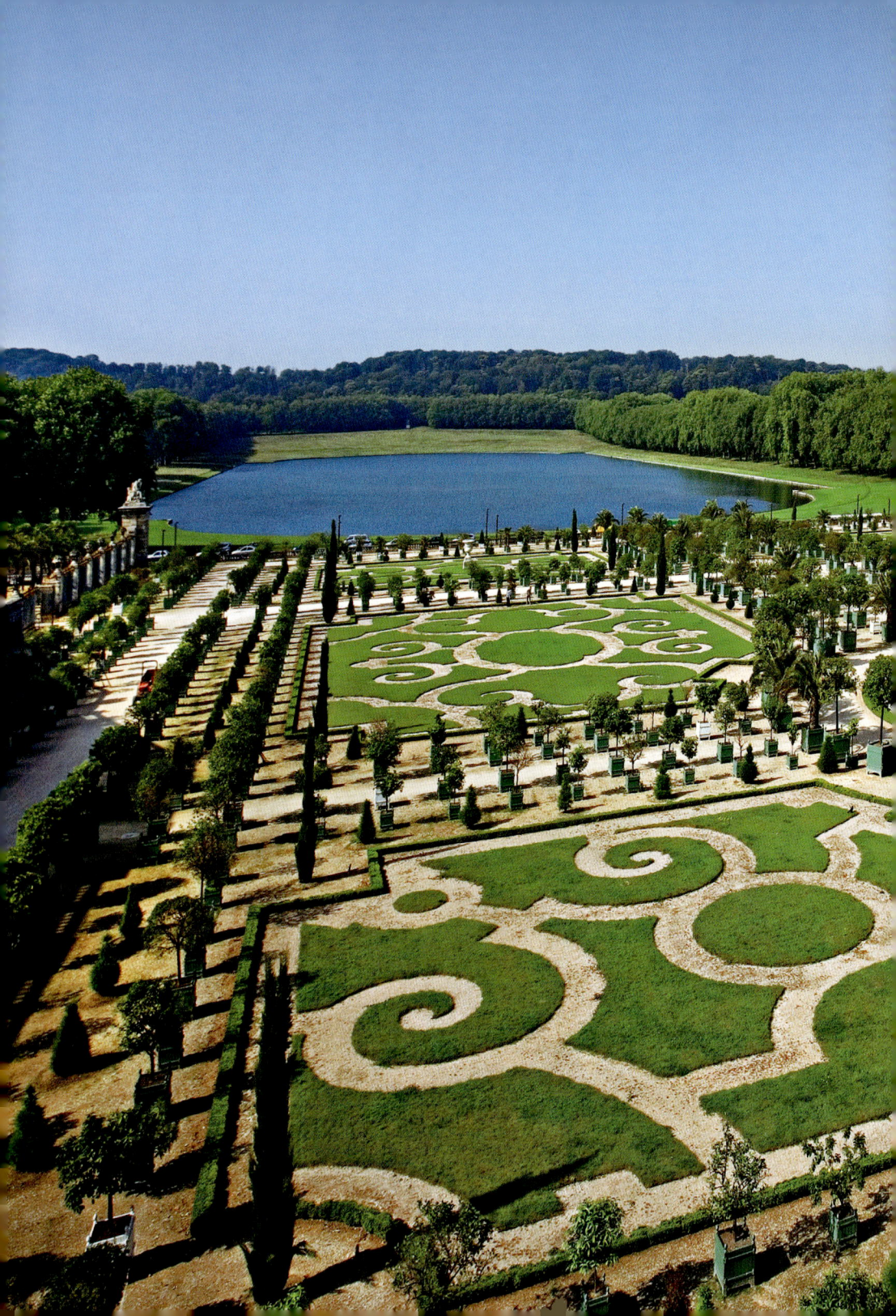

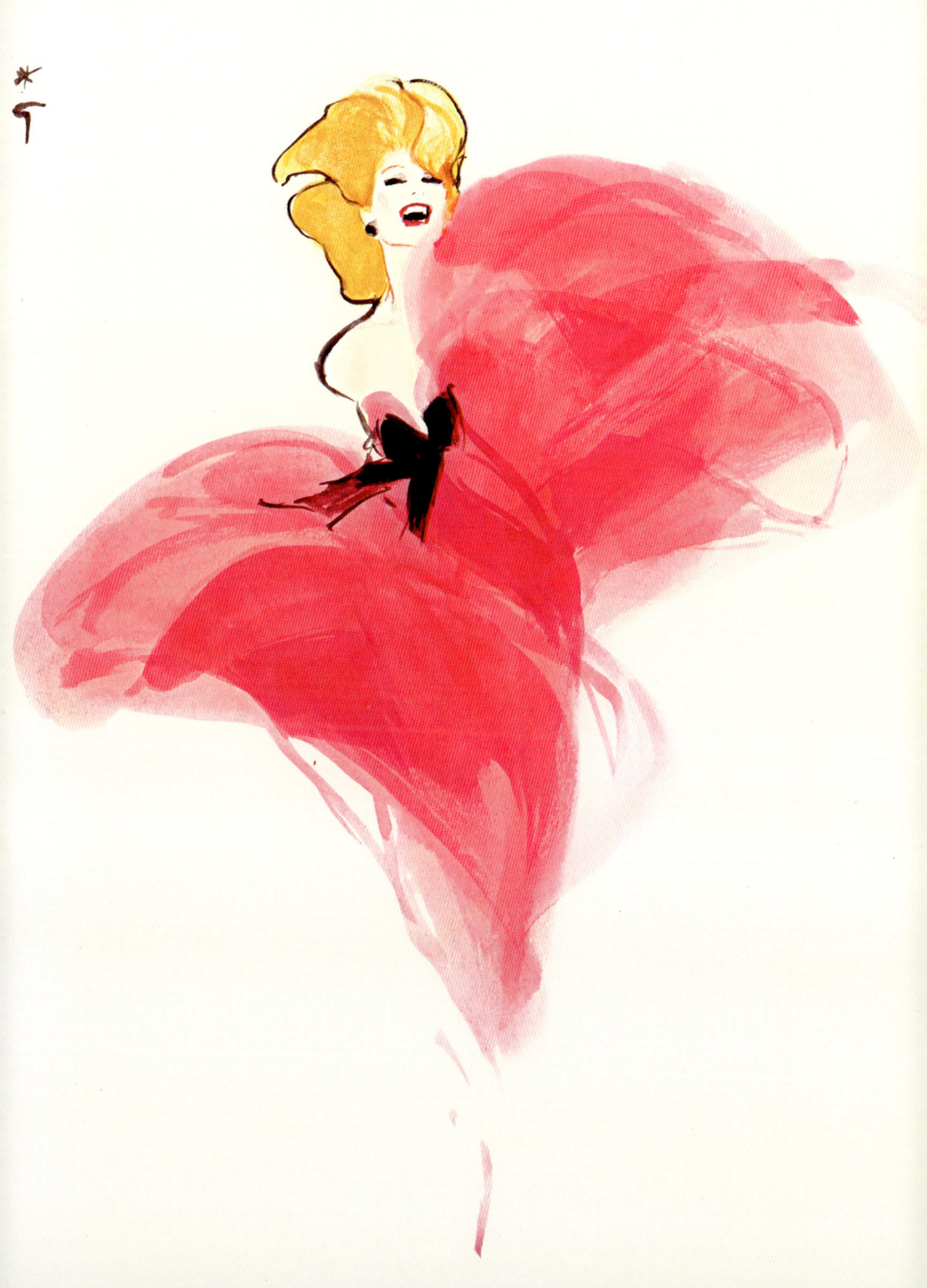

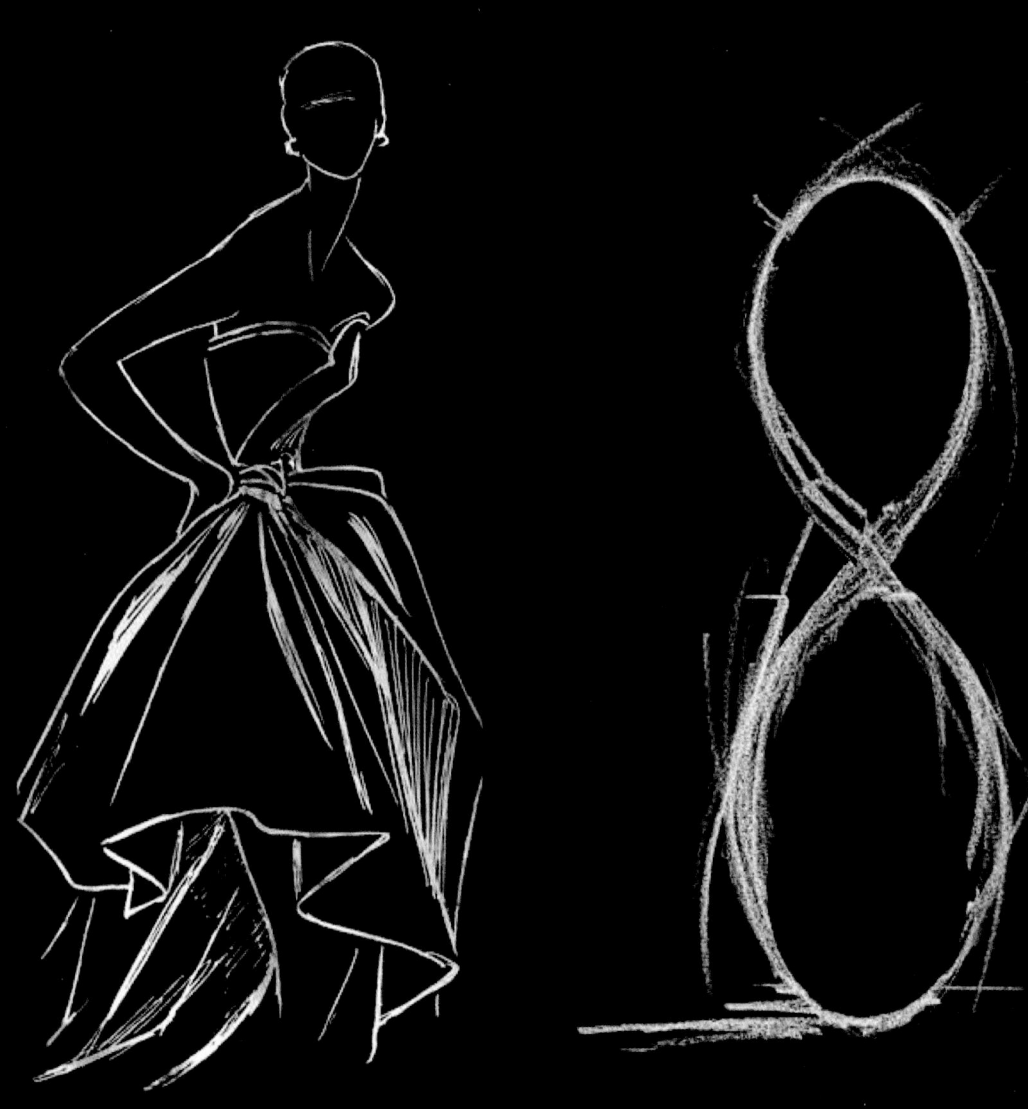

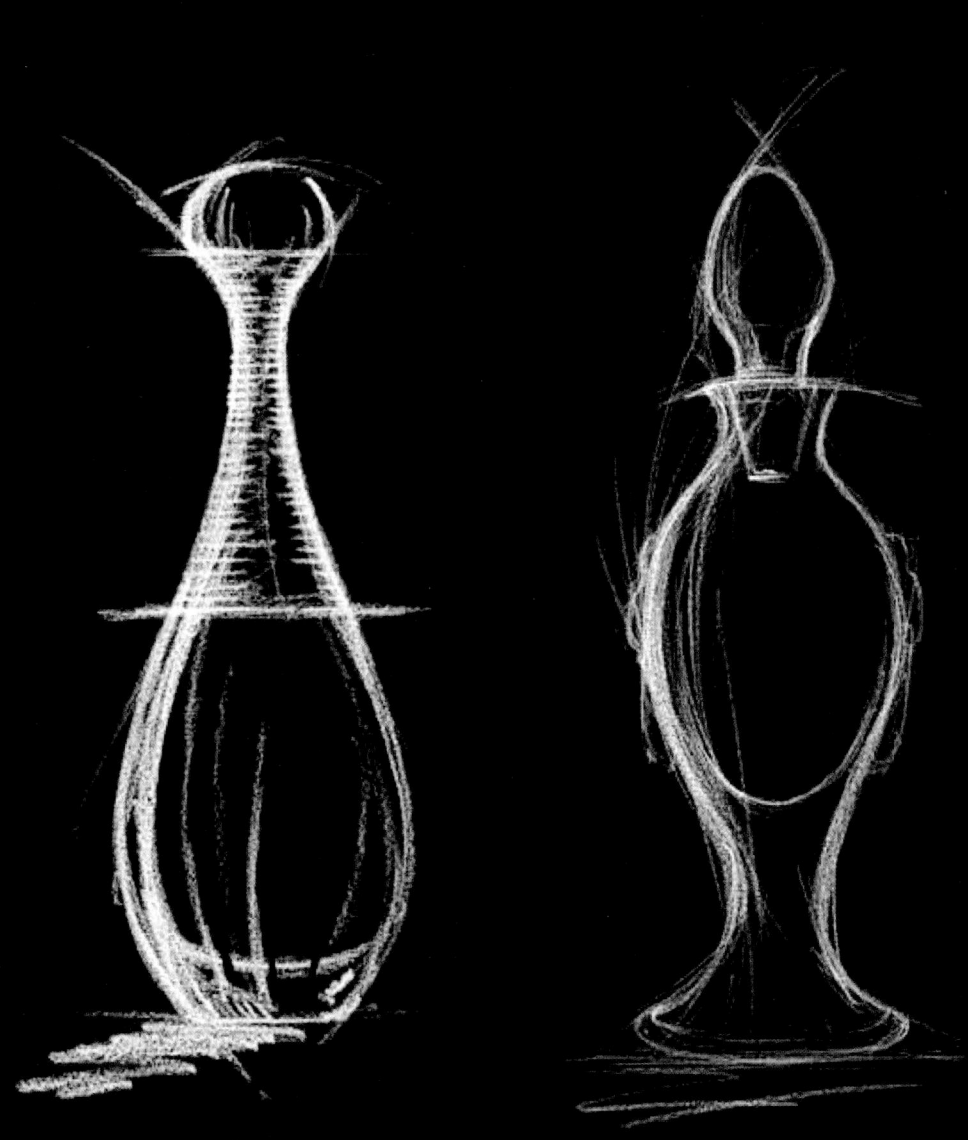

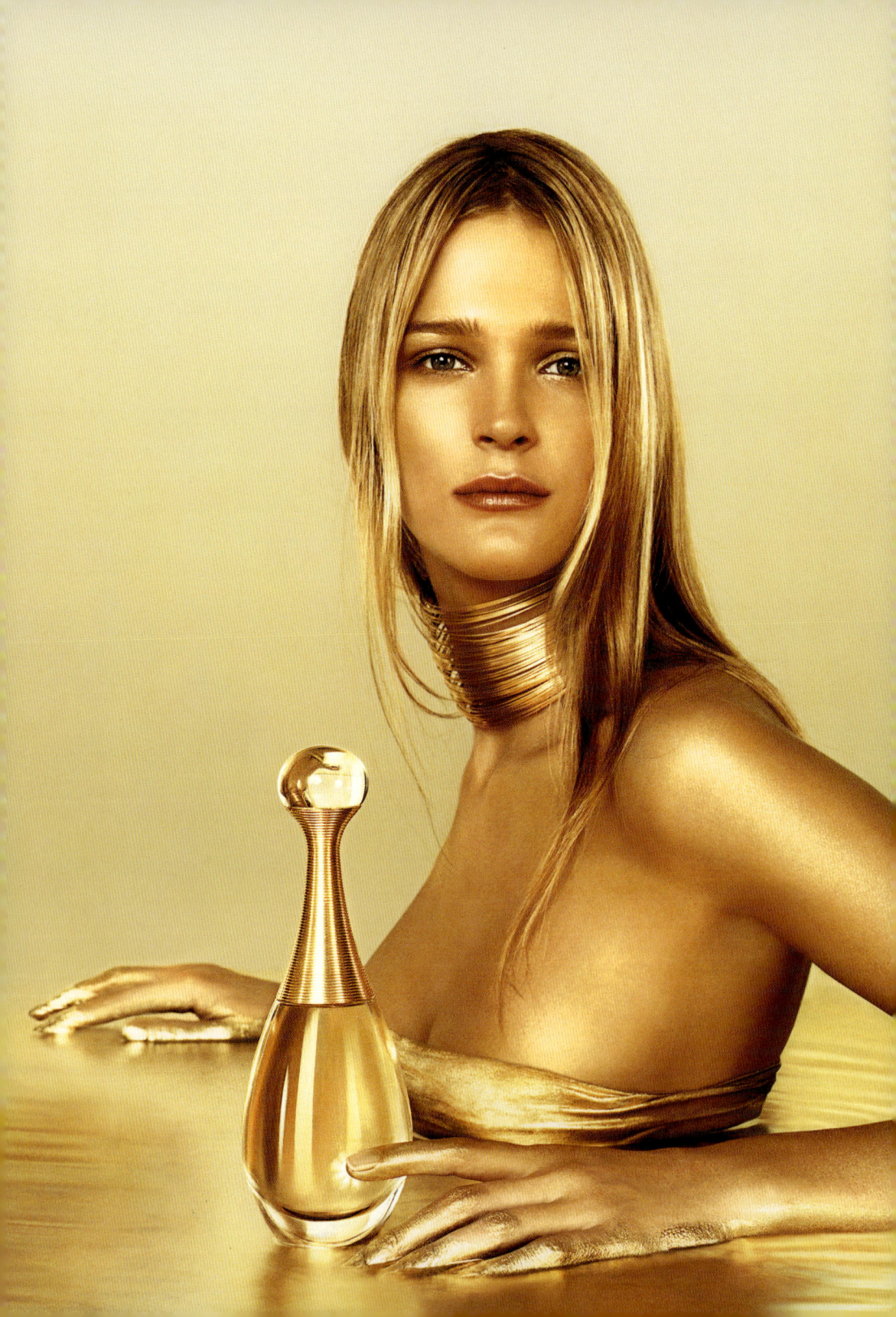

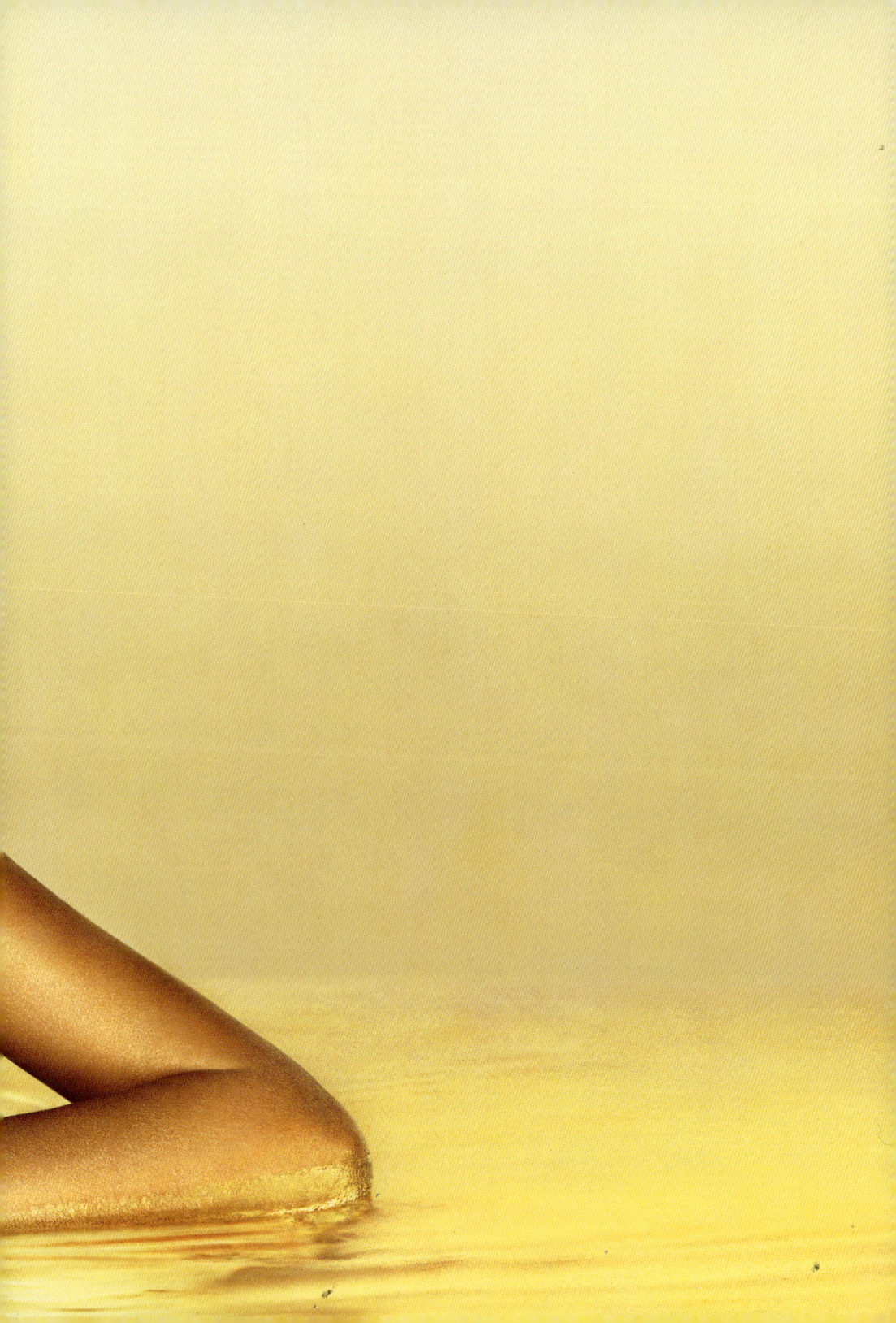

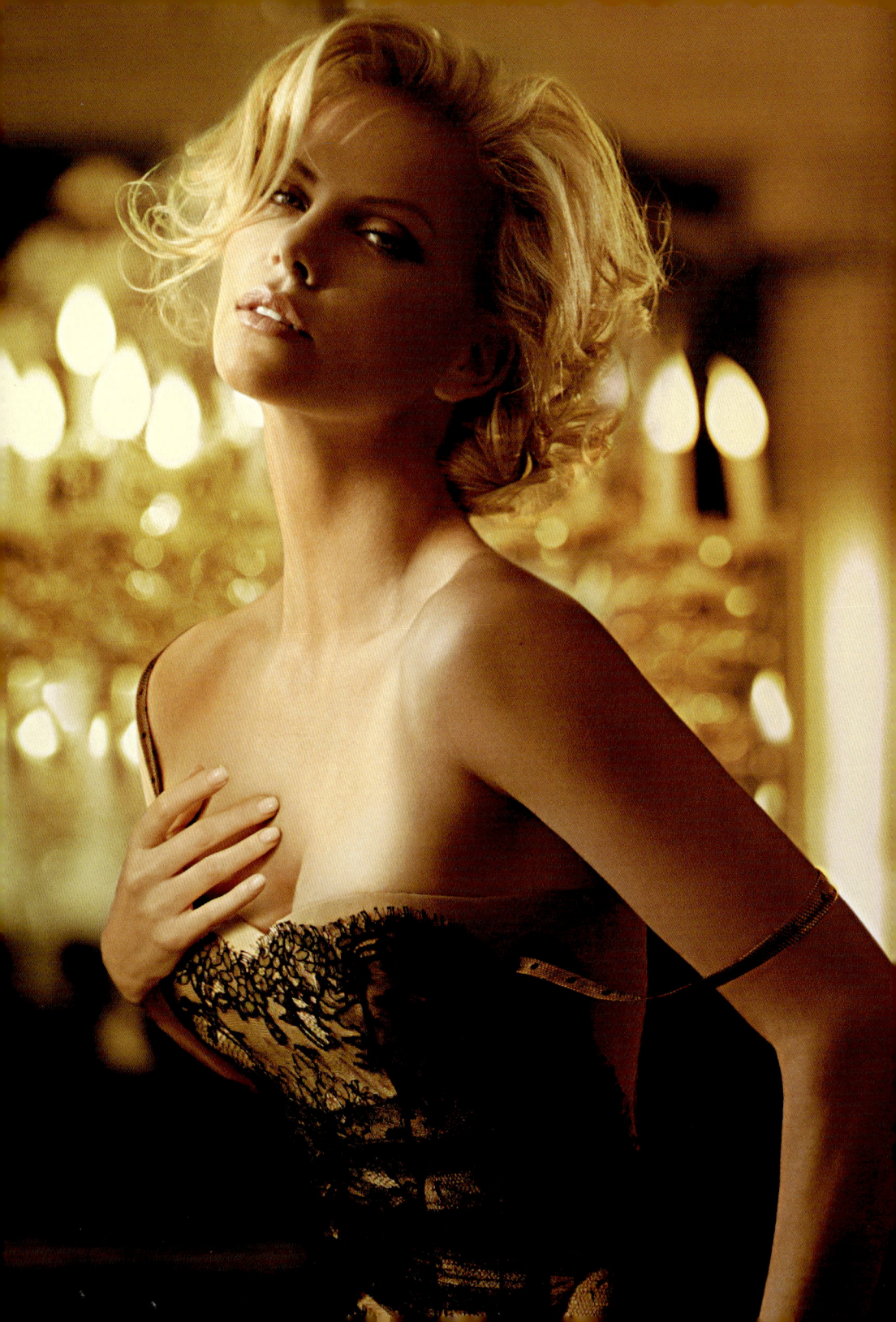

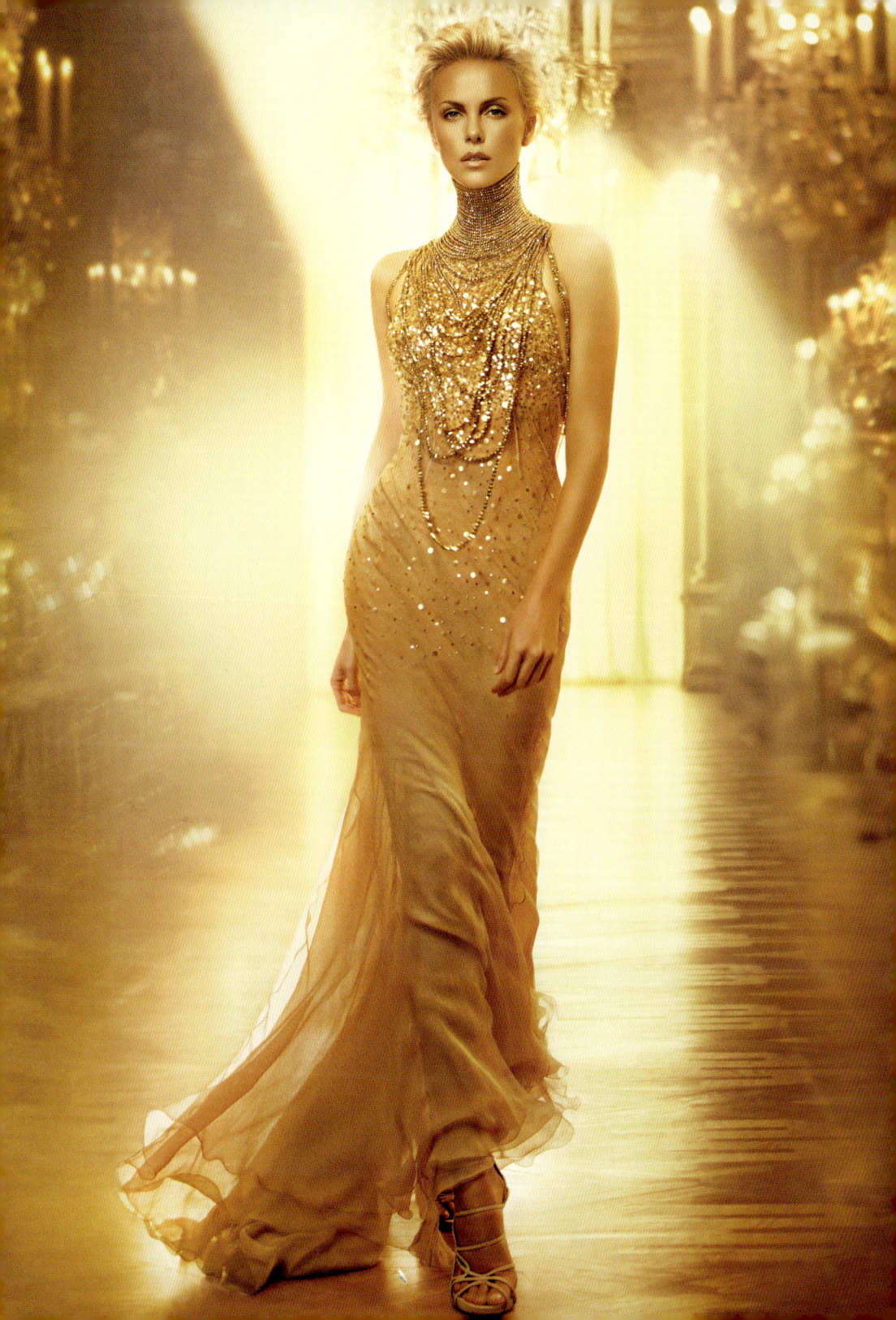

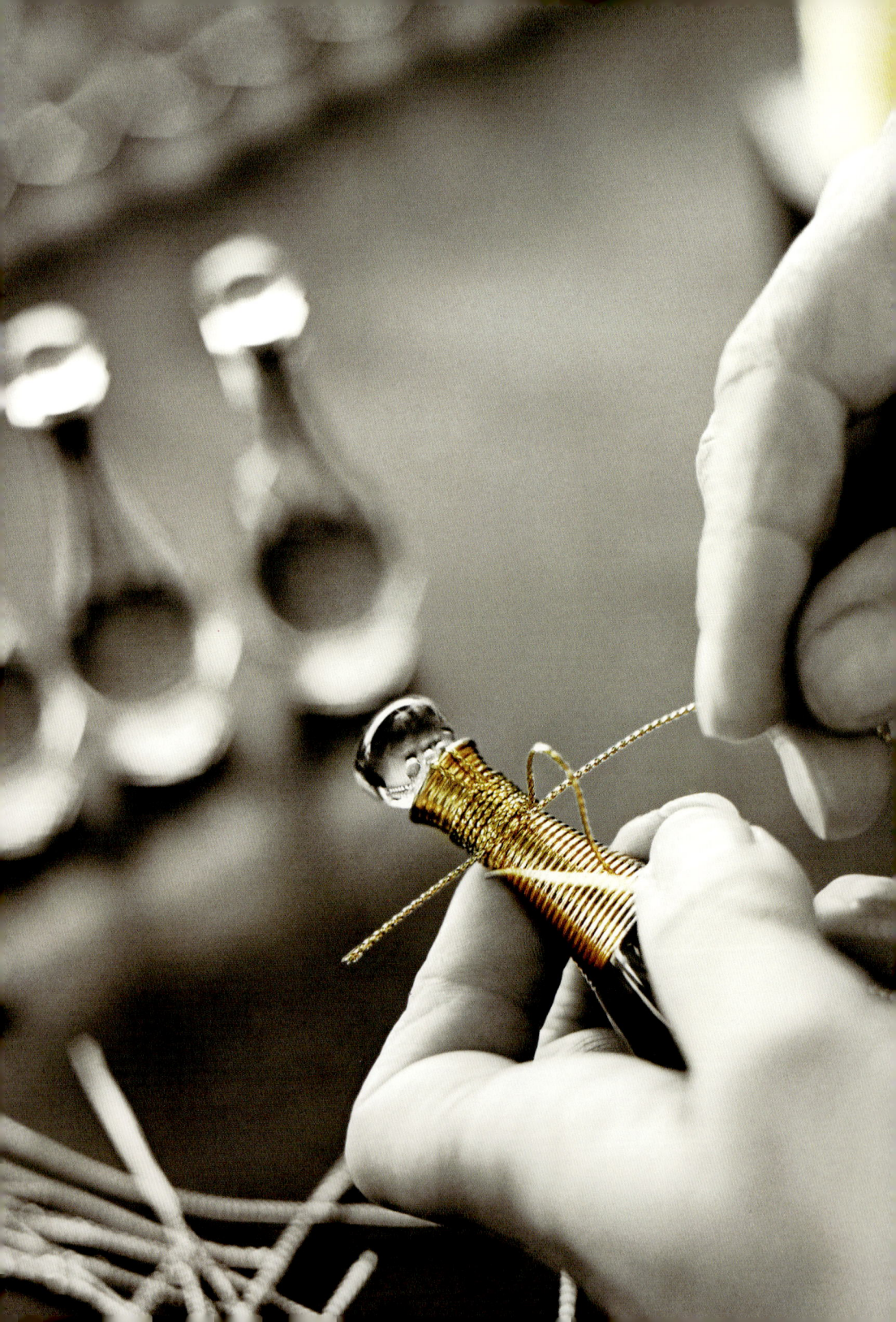

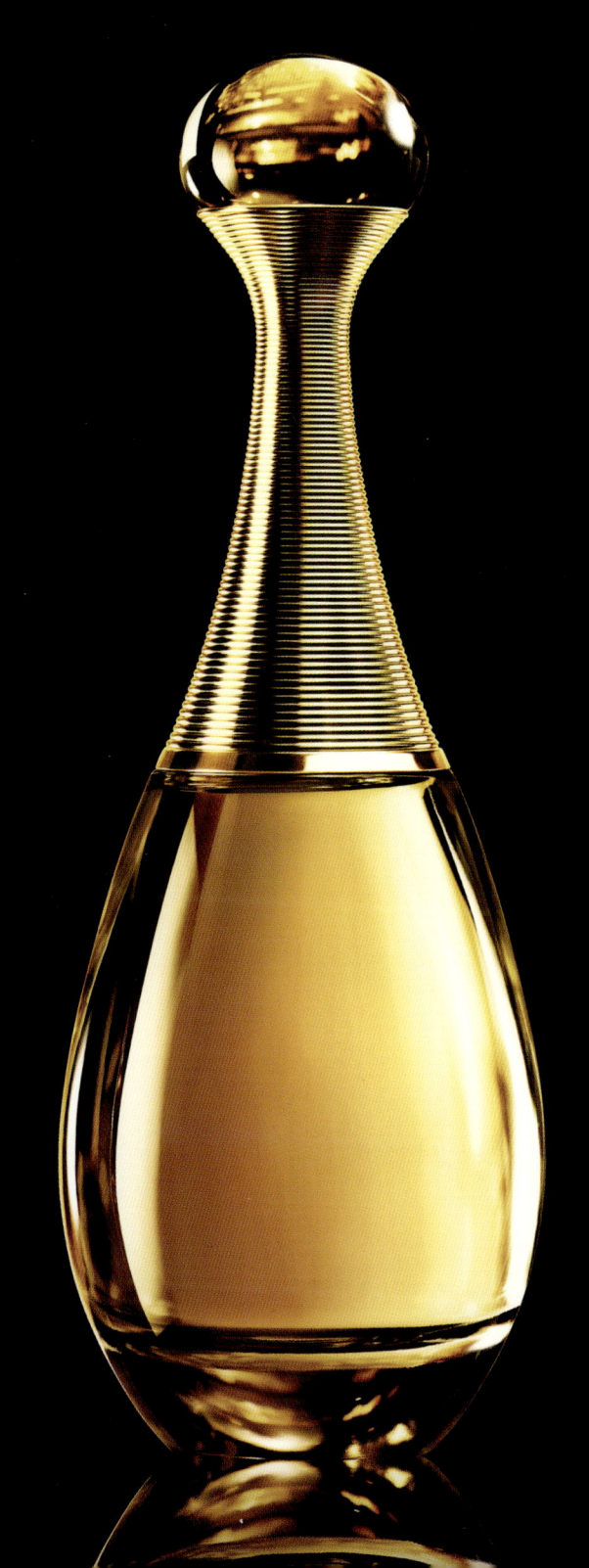

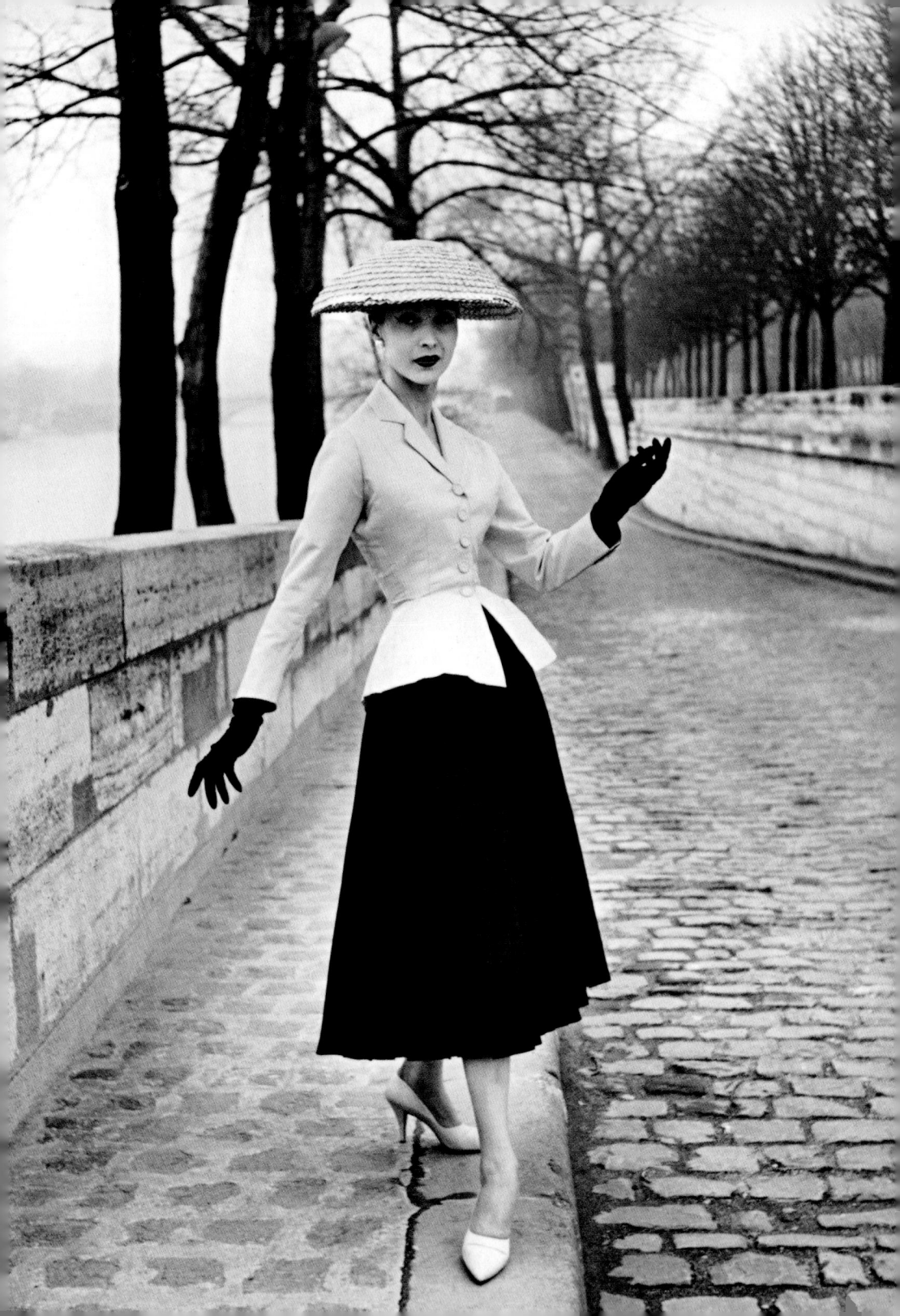

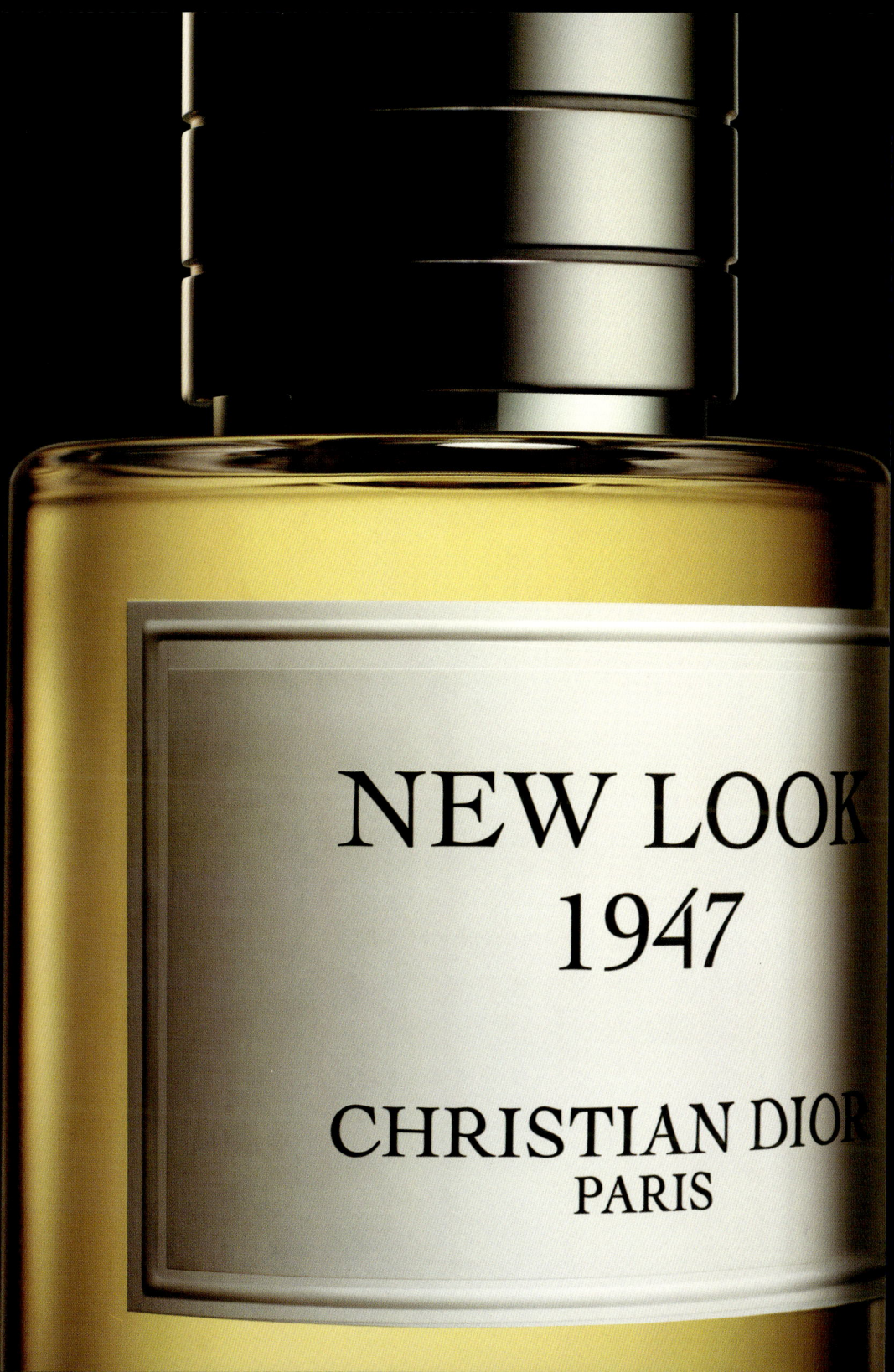

Christian Dior

présente

"Miss Dior"

son premier parfum

exclusivement en son Hôtel, 30 Avenue Montaigne

à partir du 17 Décembre 1947.

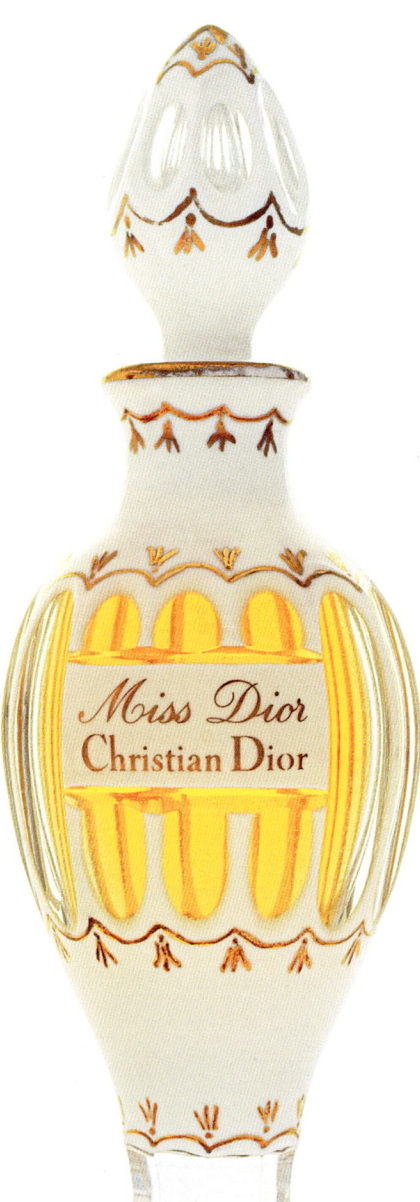

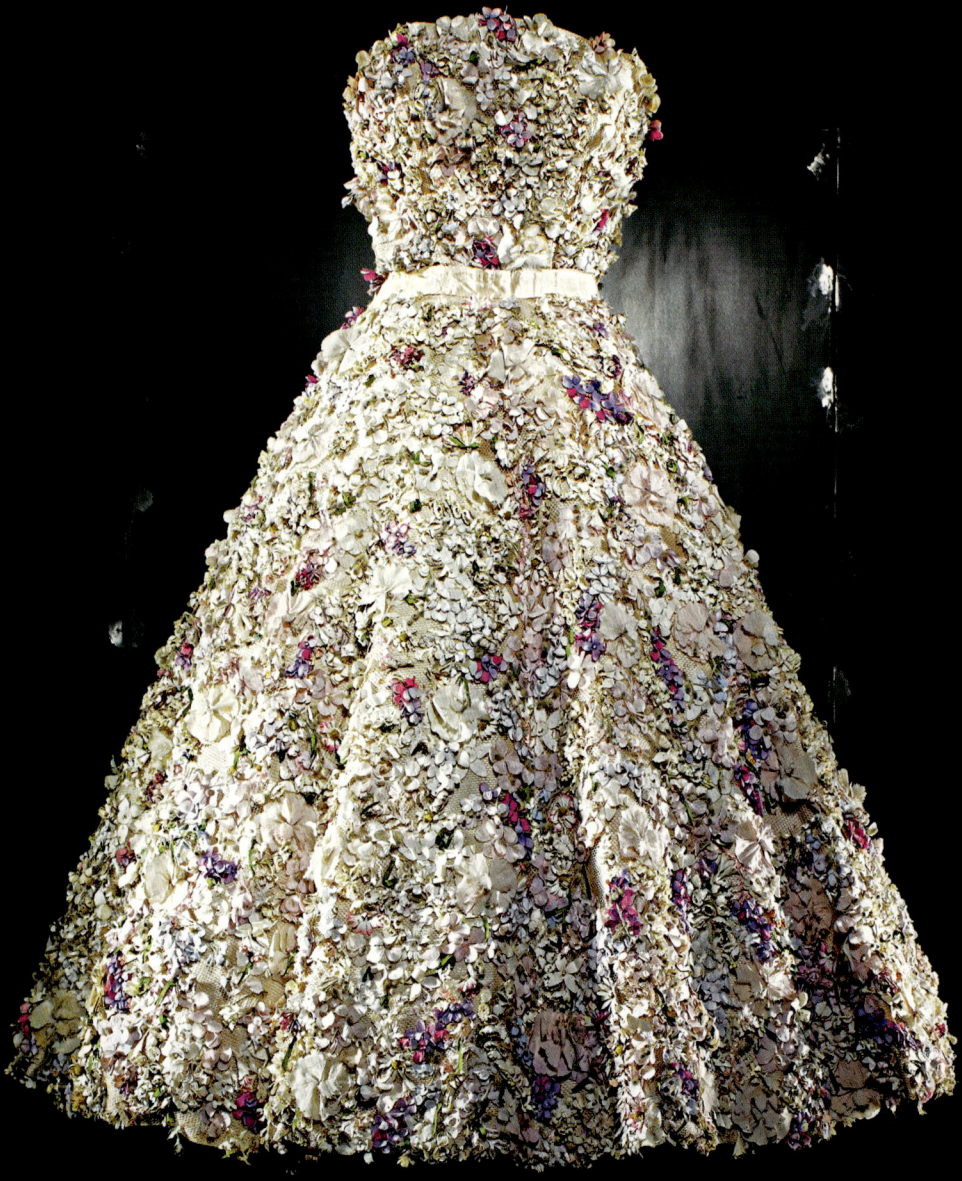

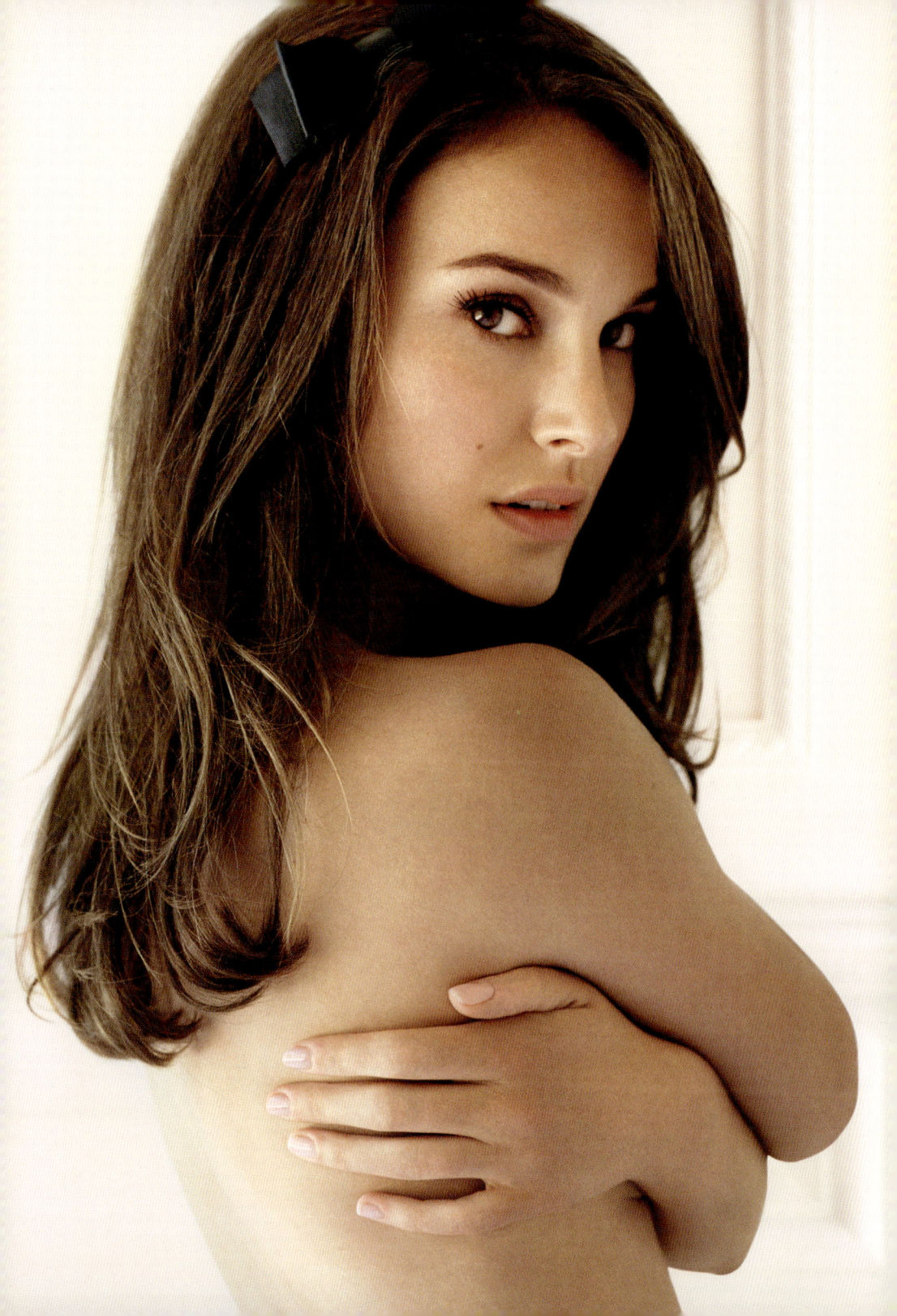

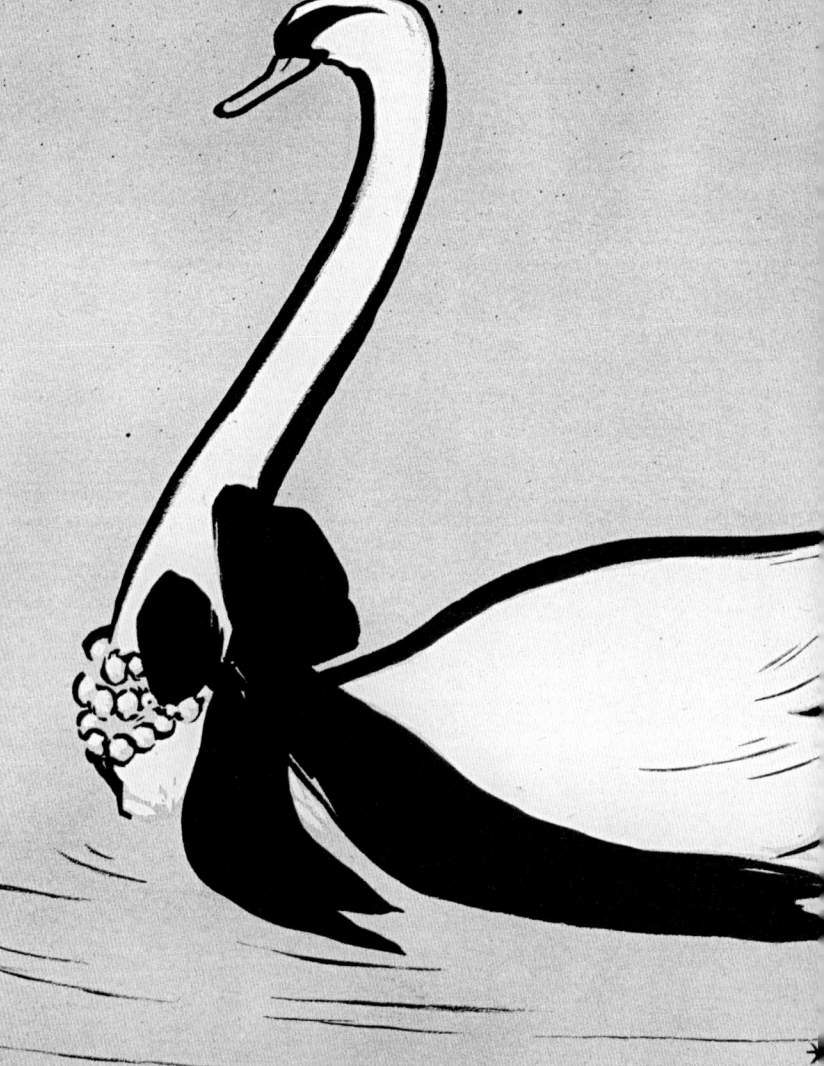

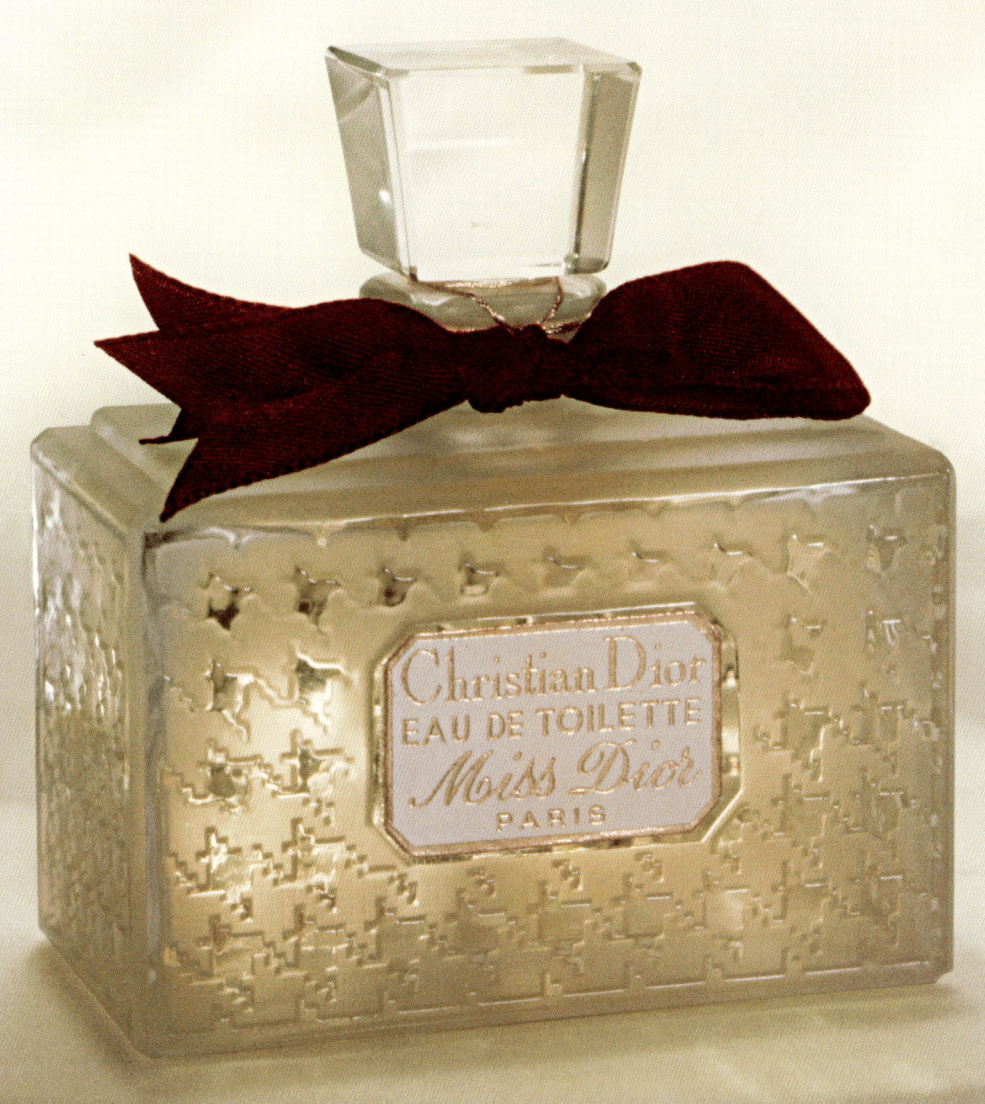

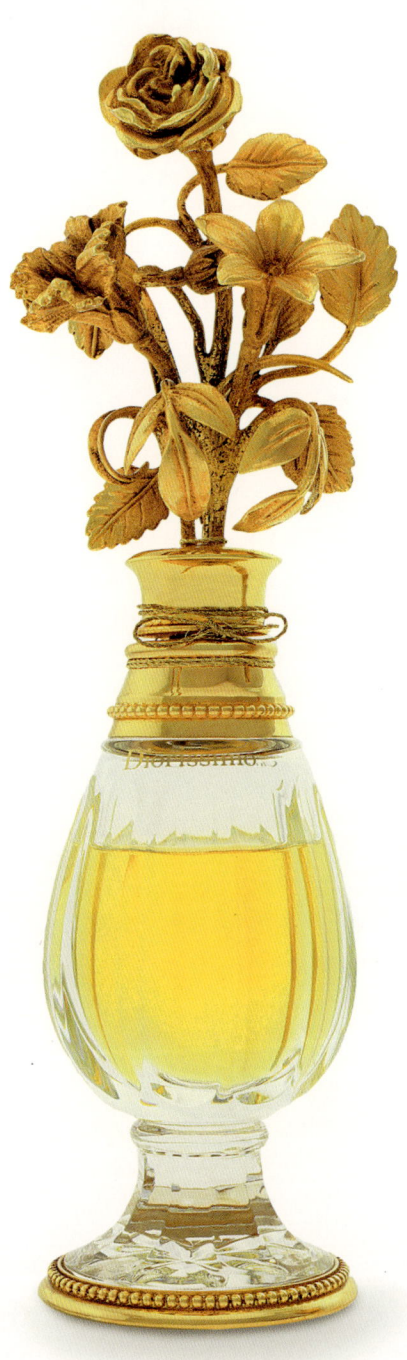

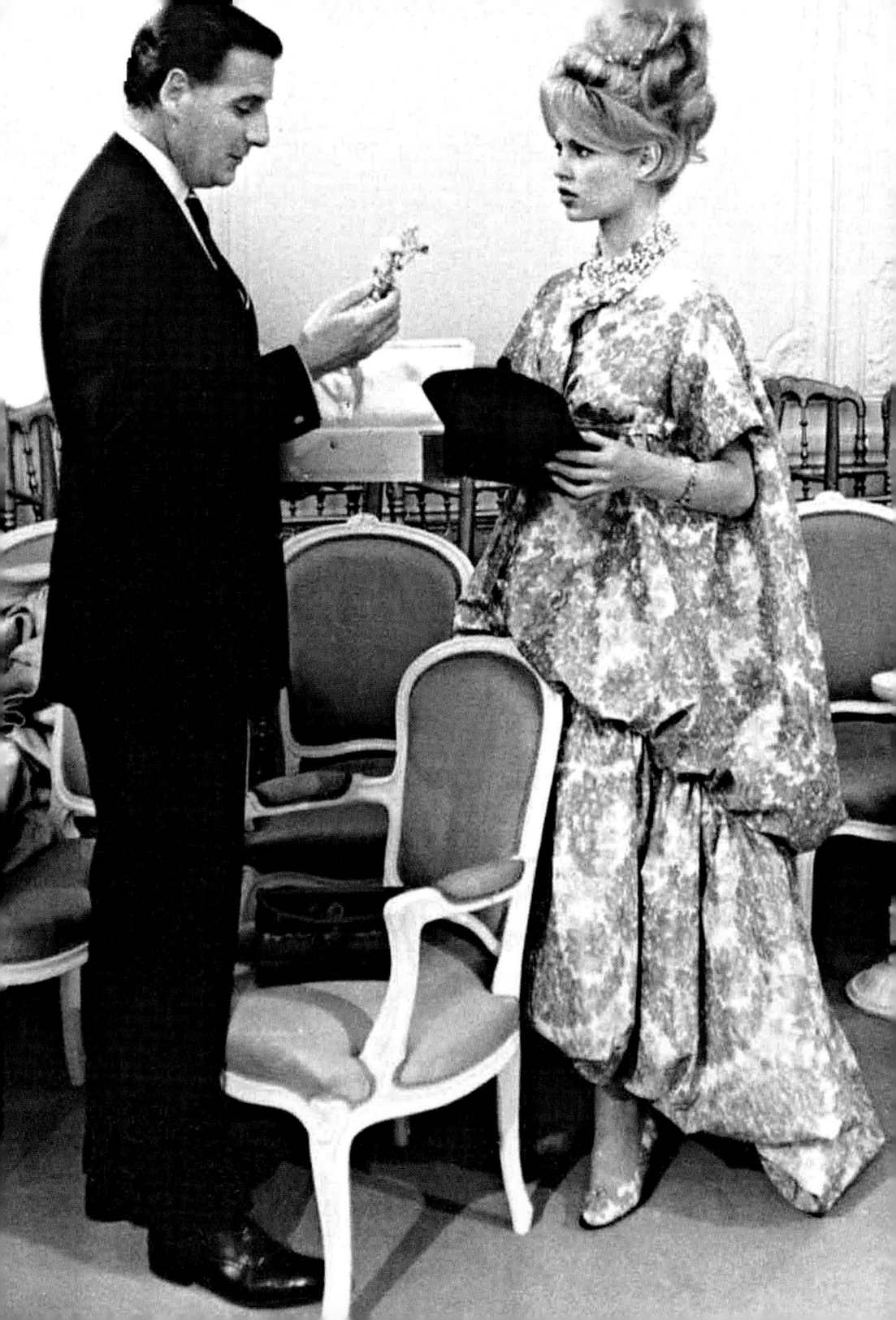

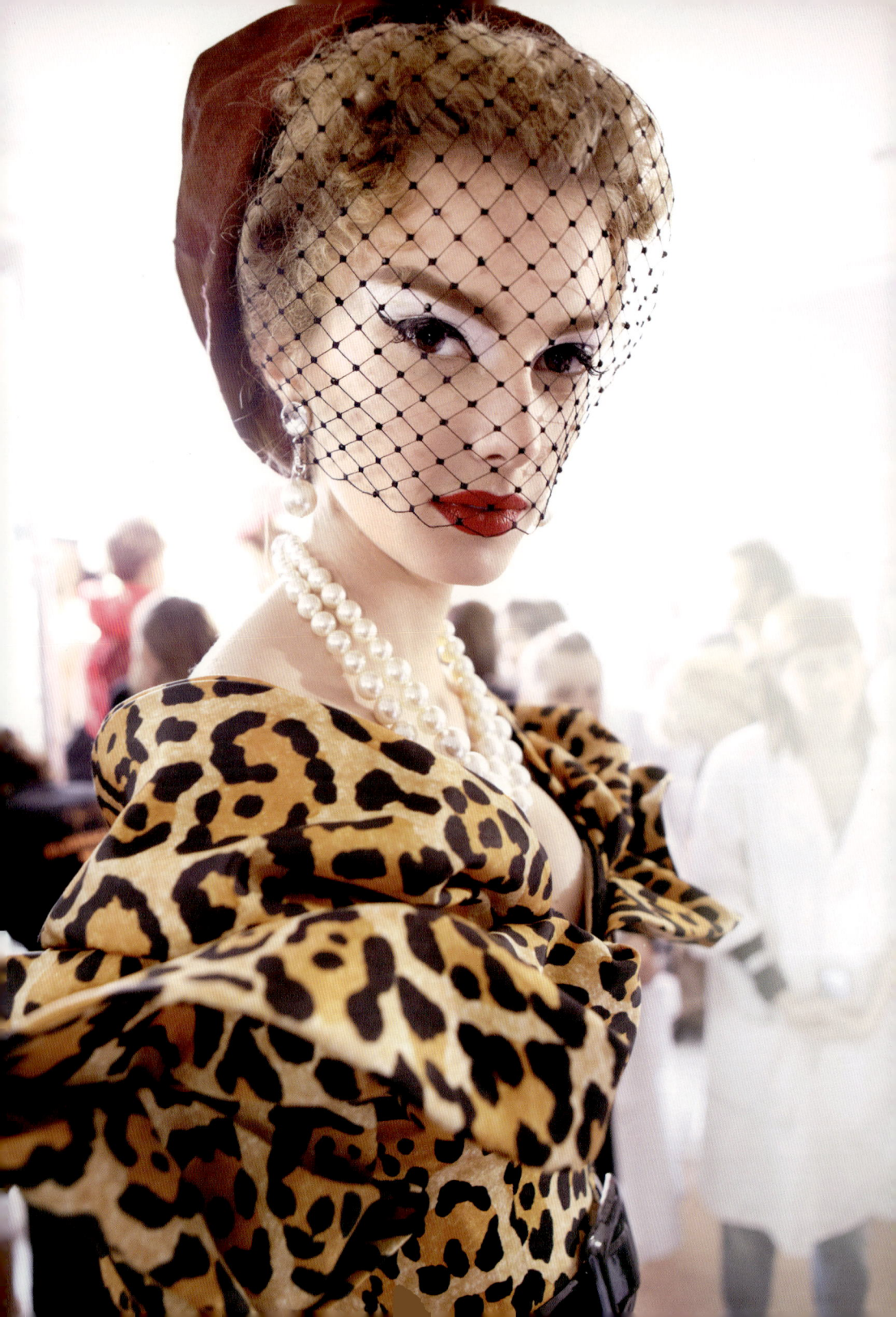

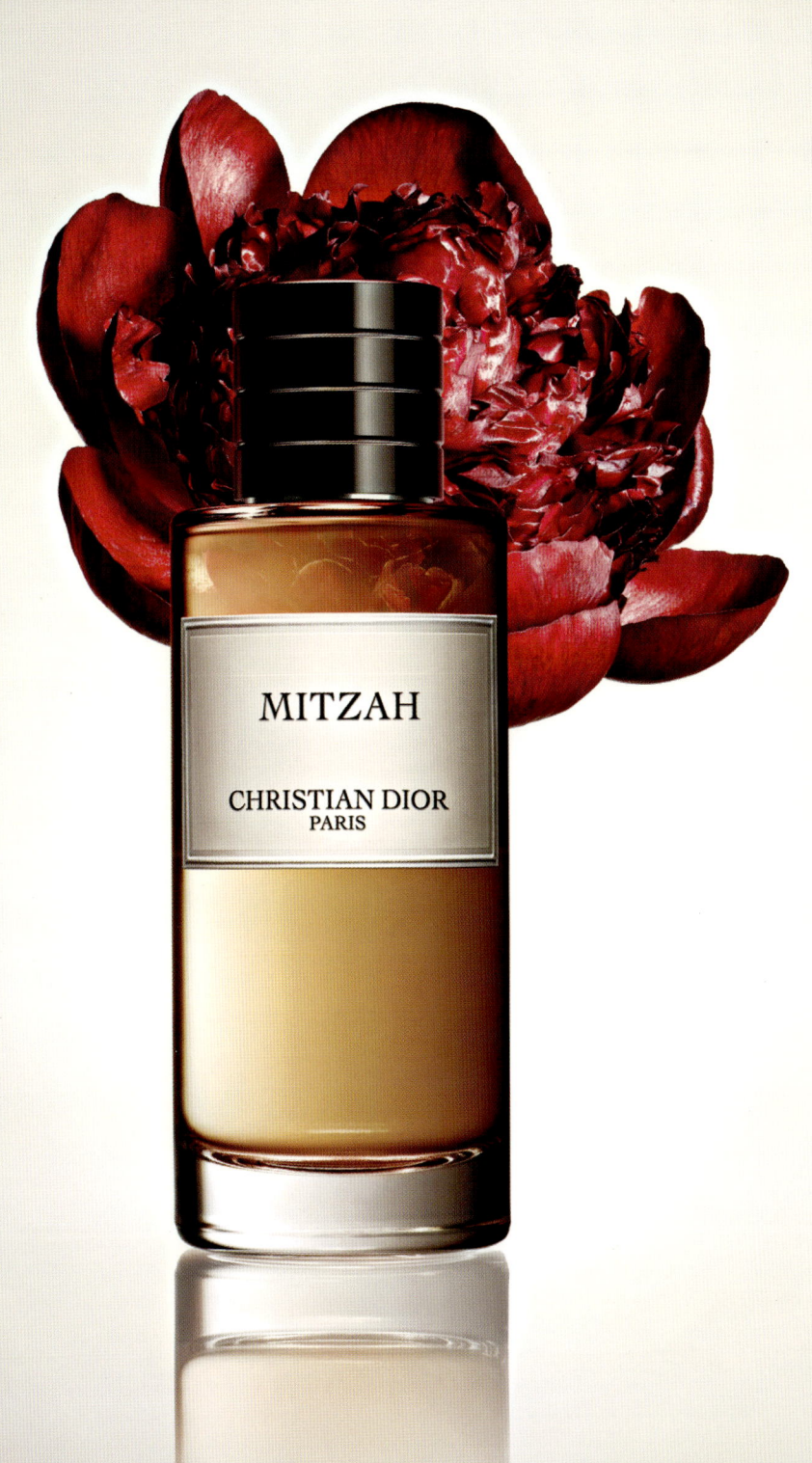

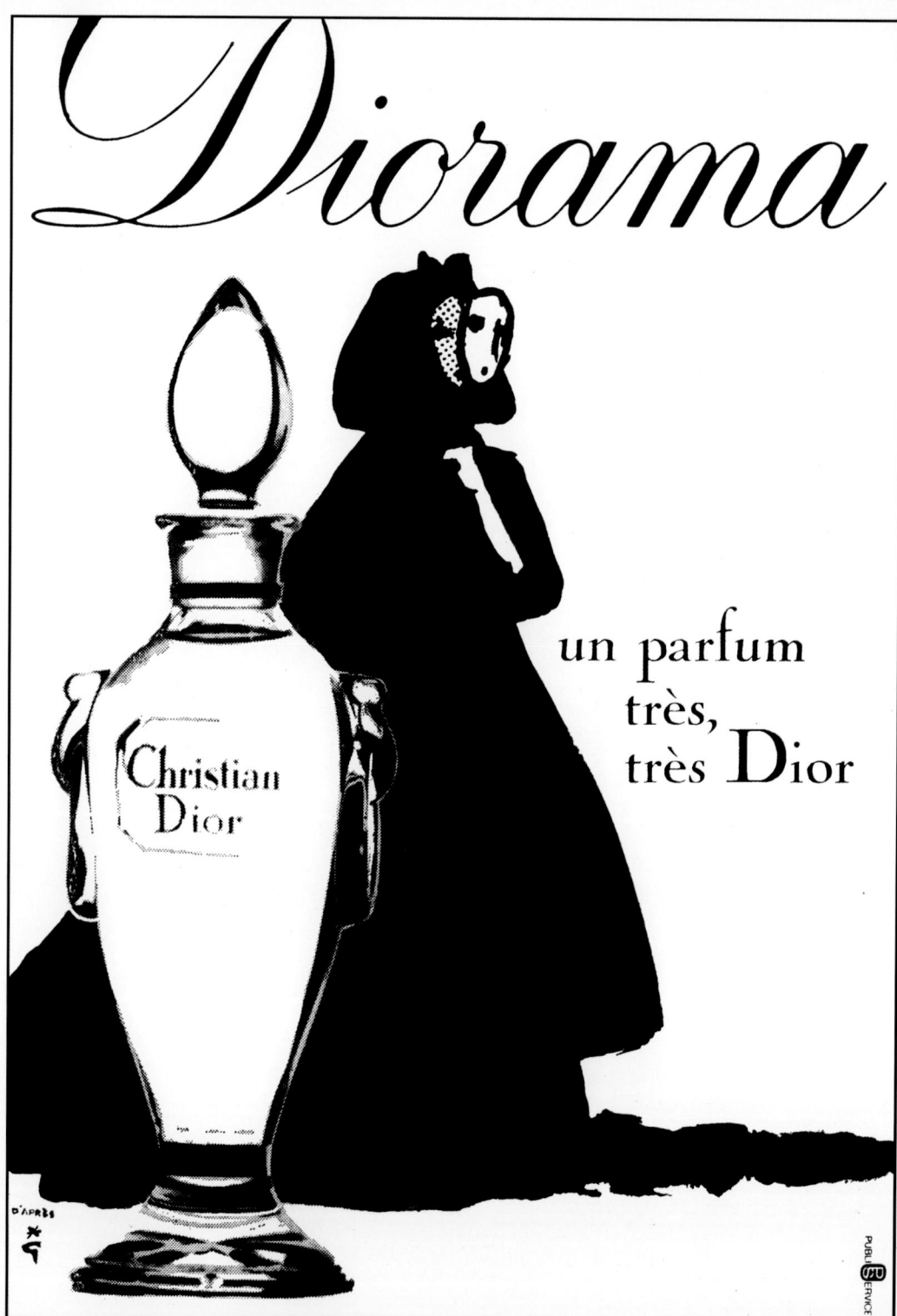

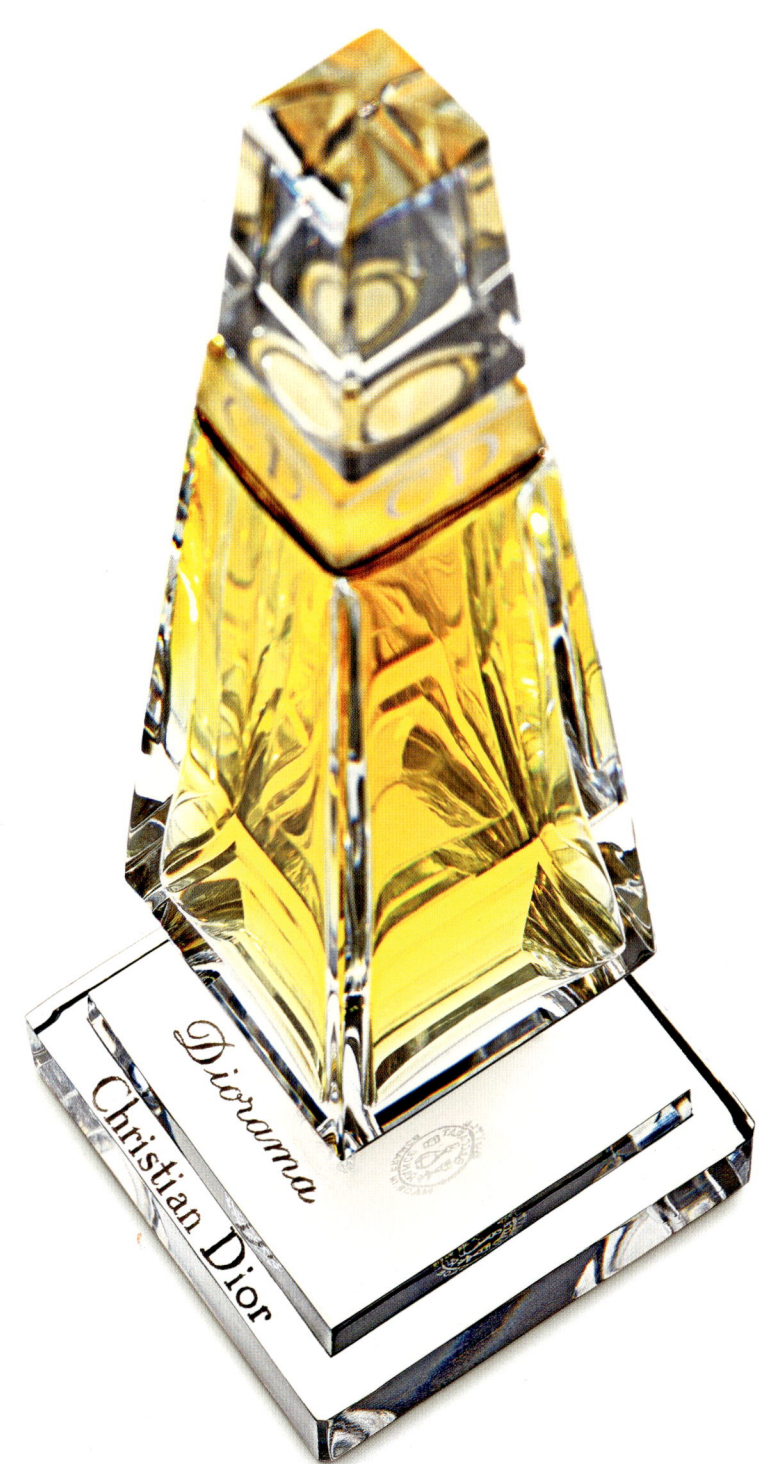

après le sport...

...l'eau fraîche de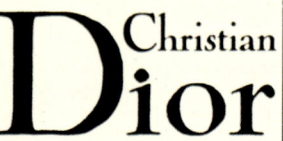

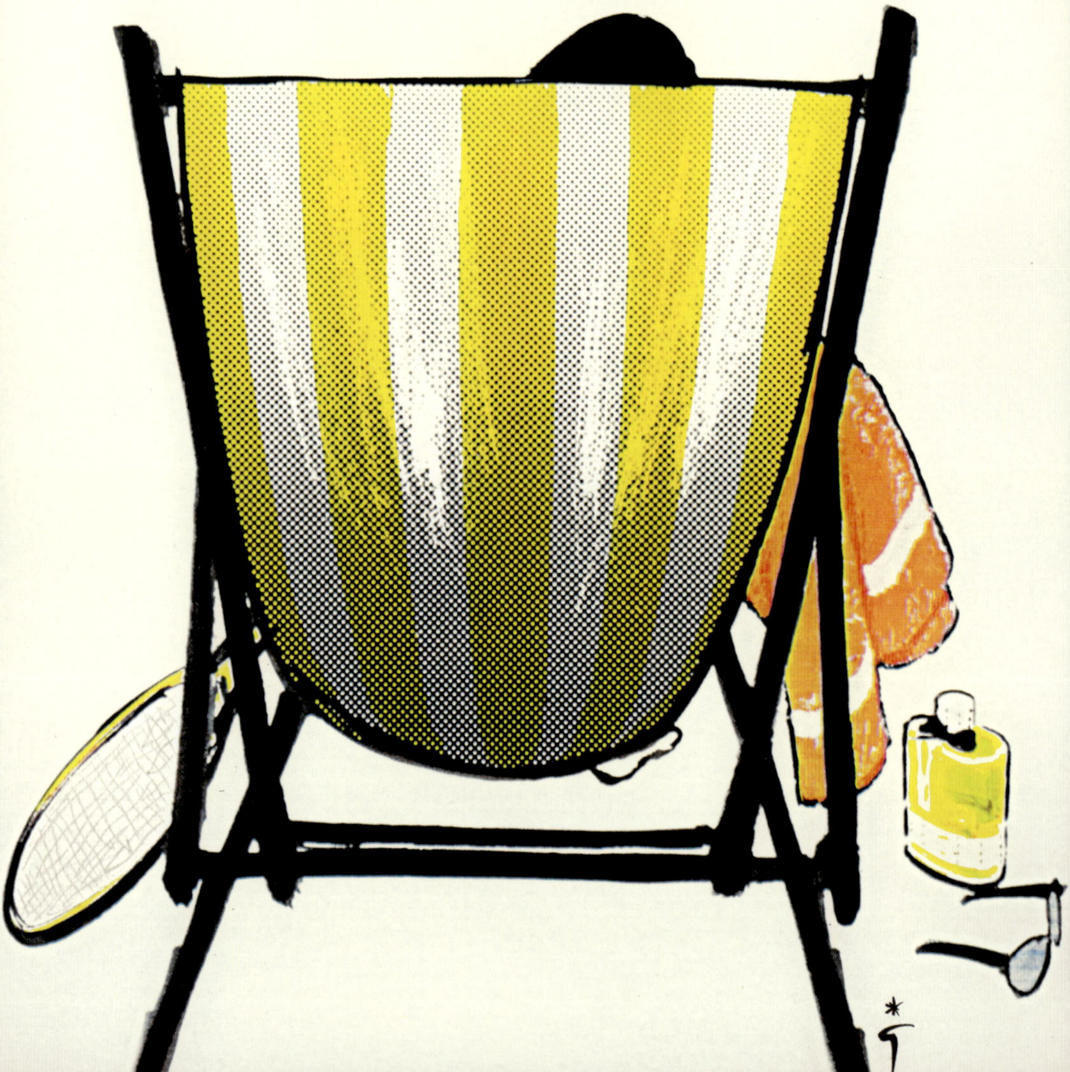

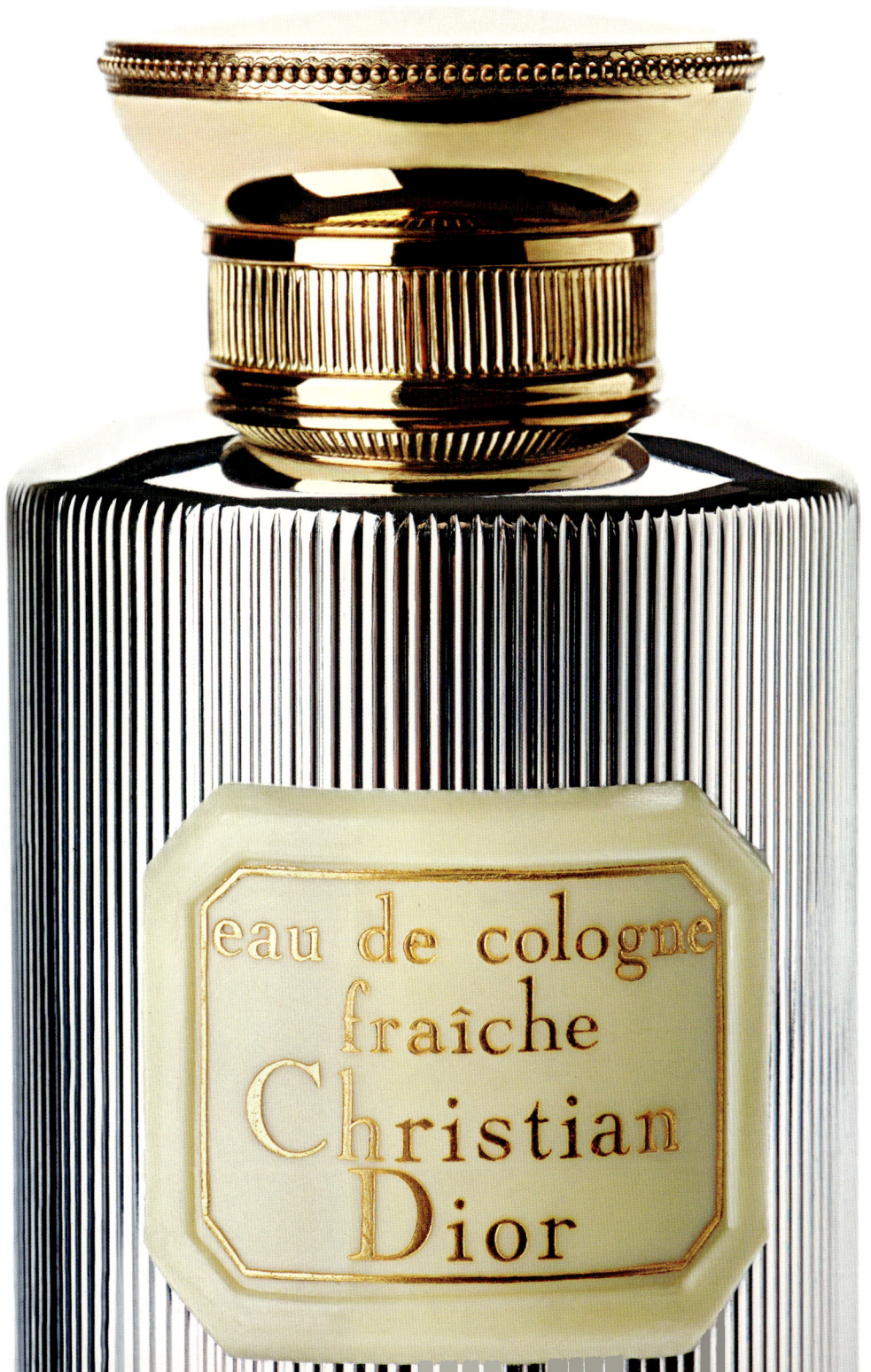

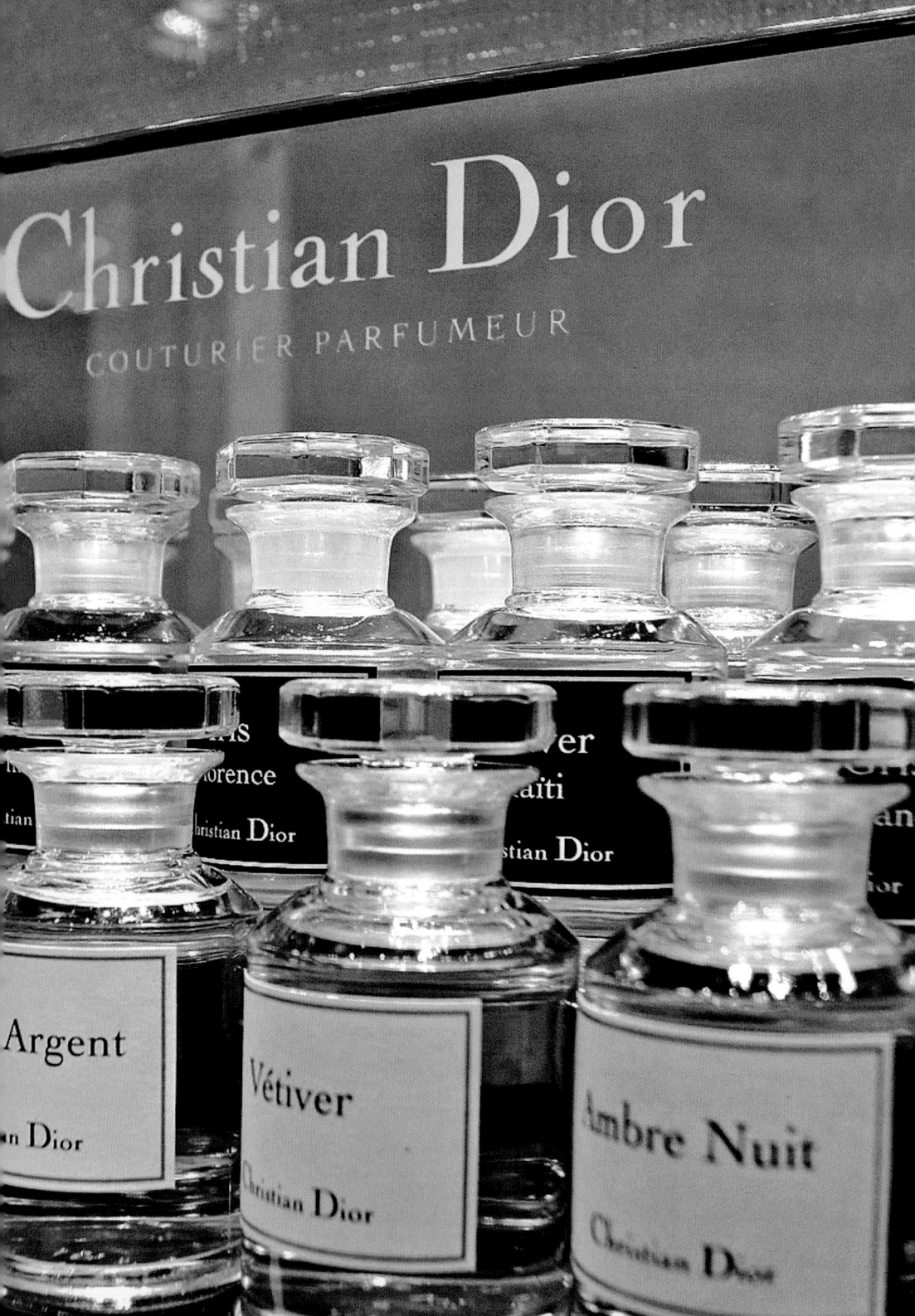

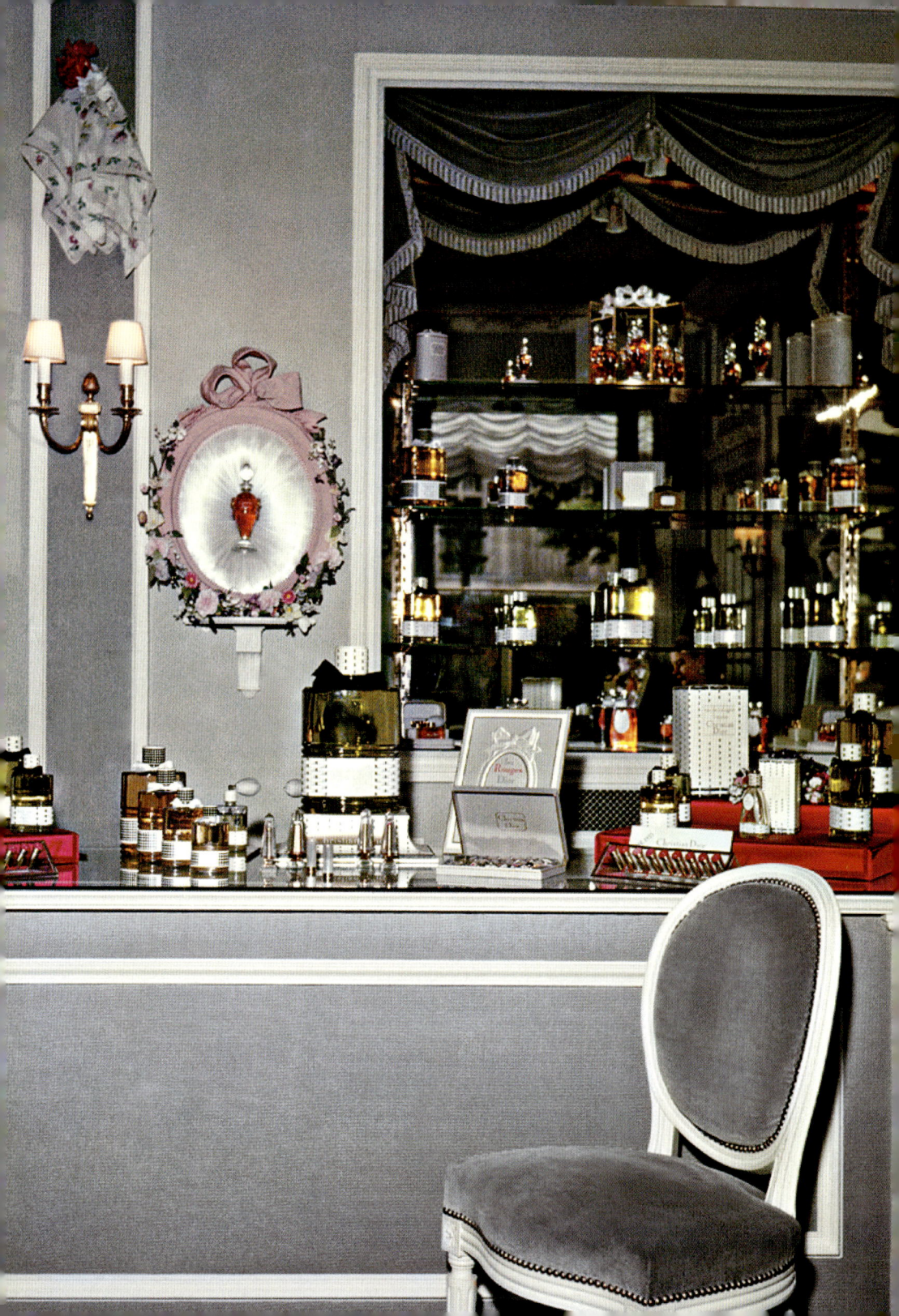

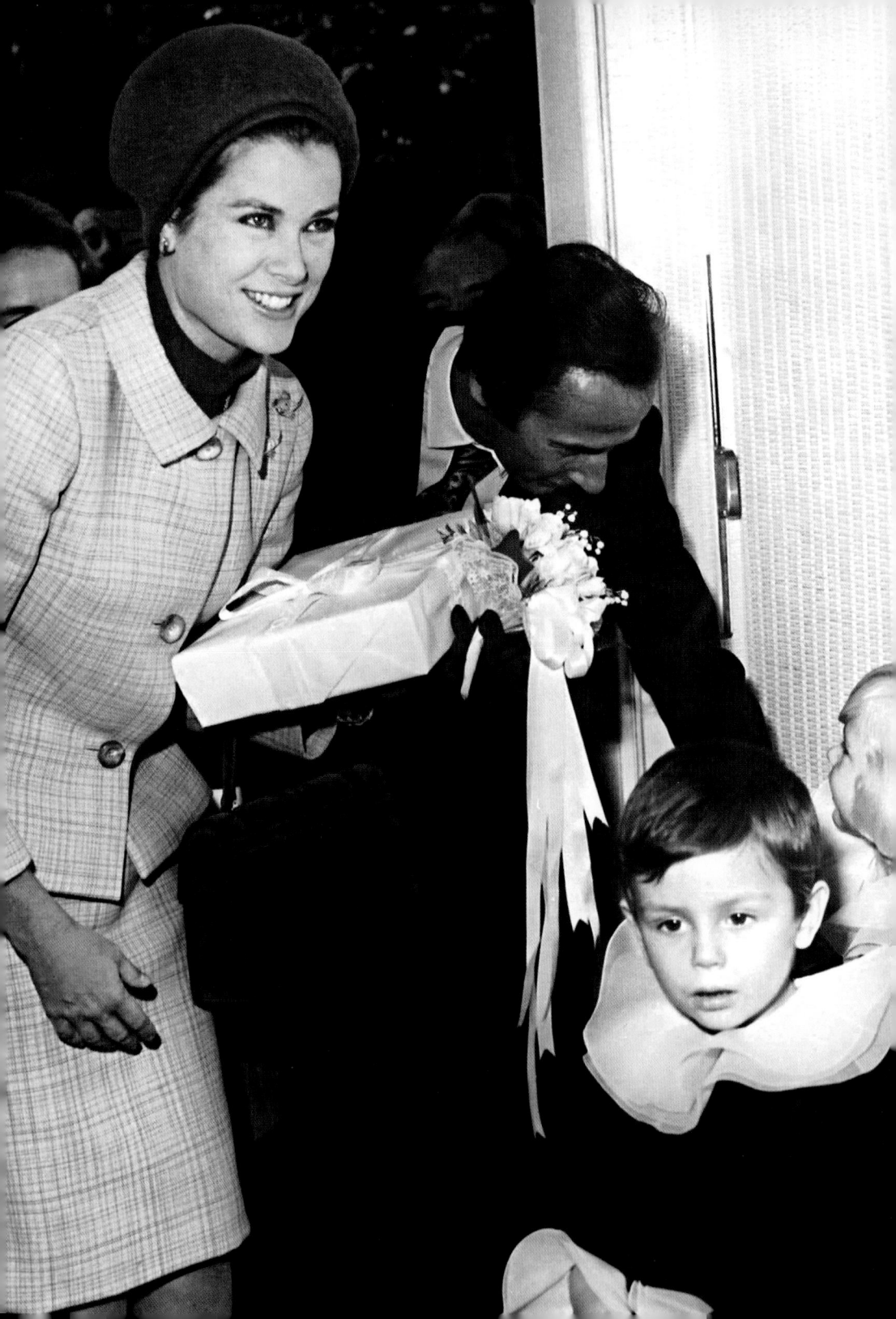

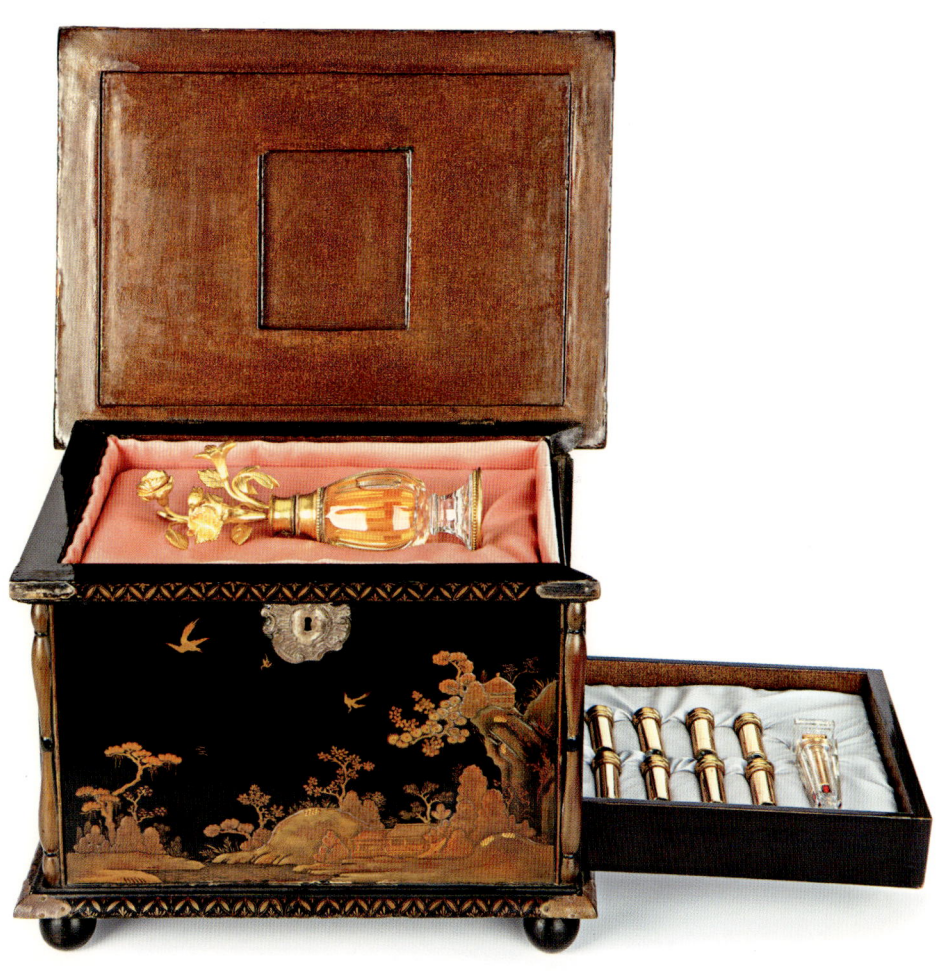

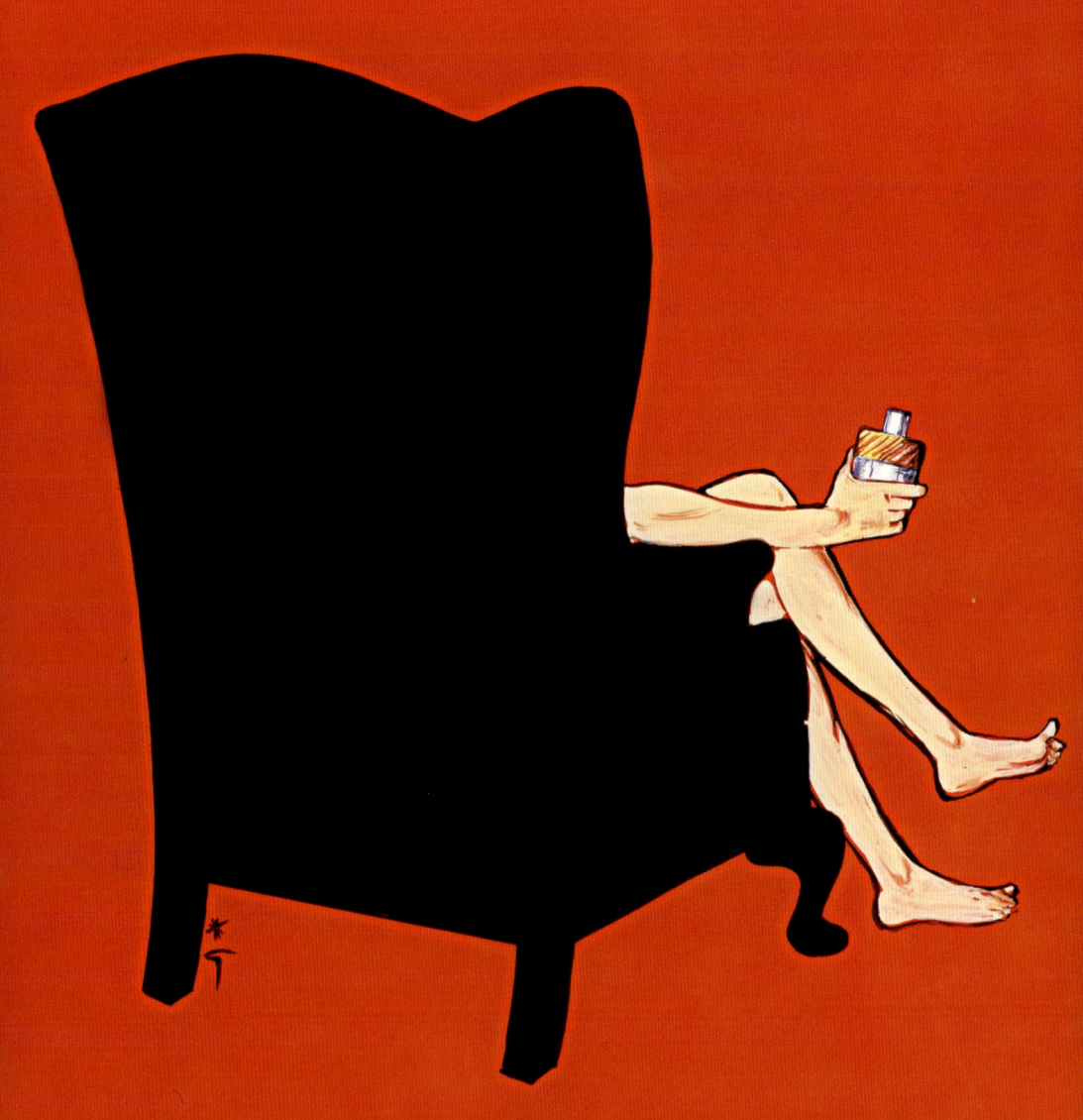

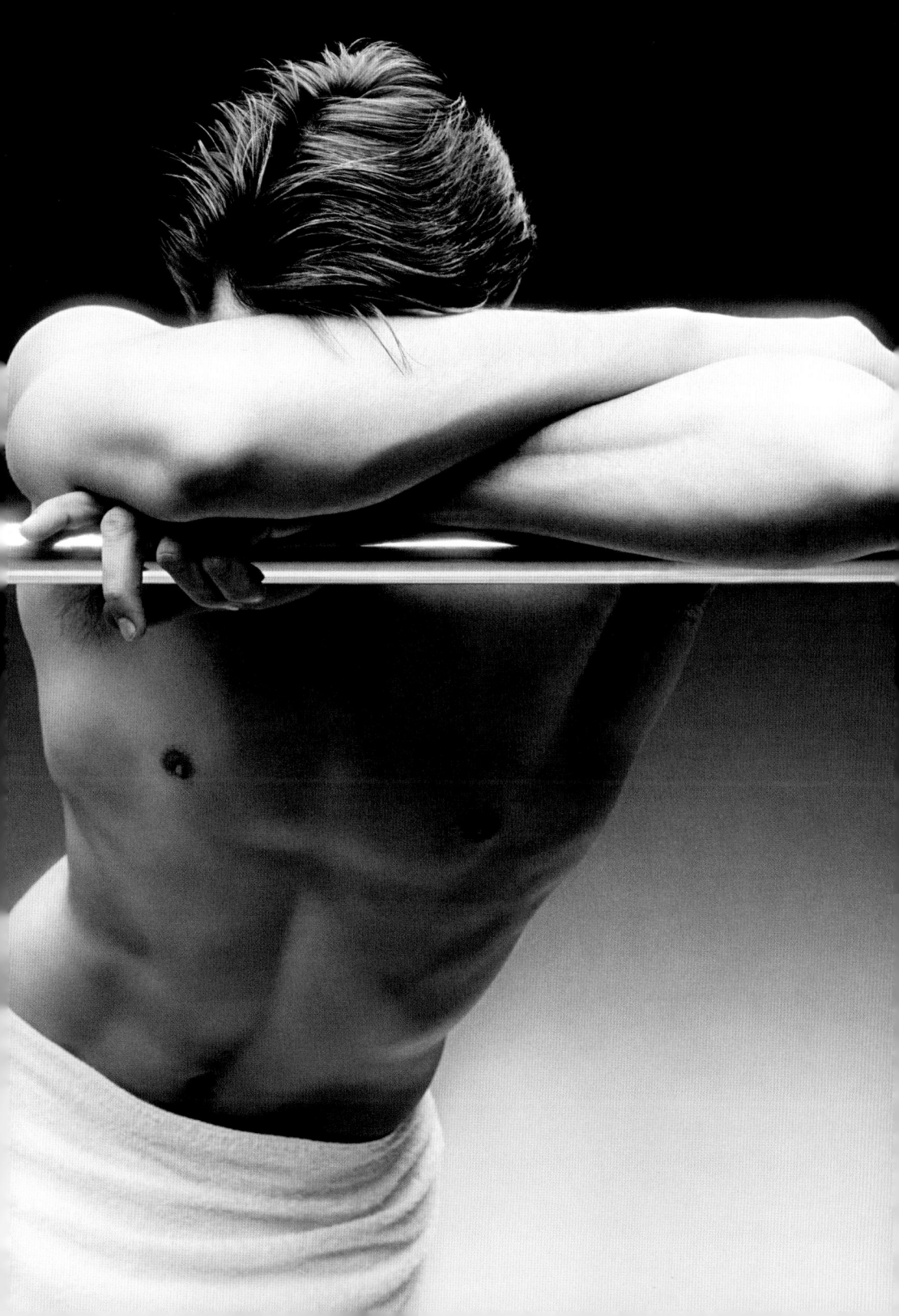

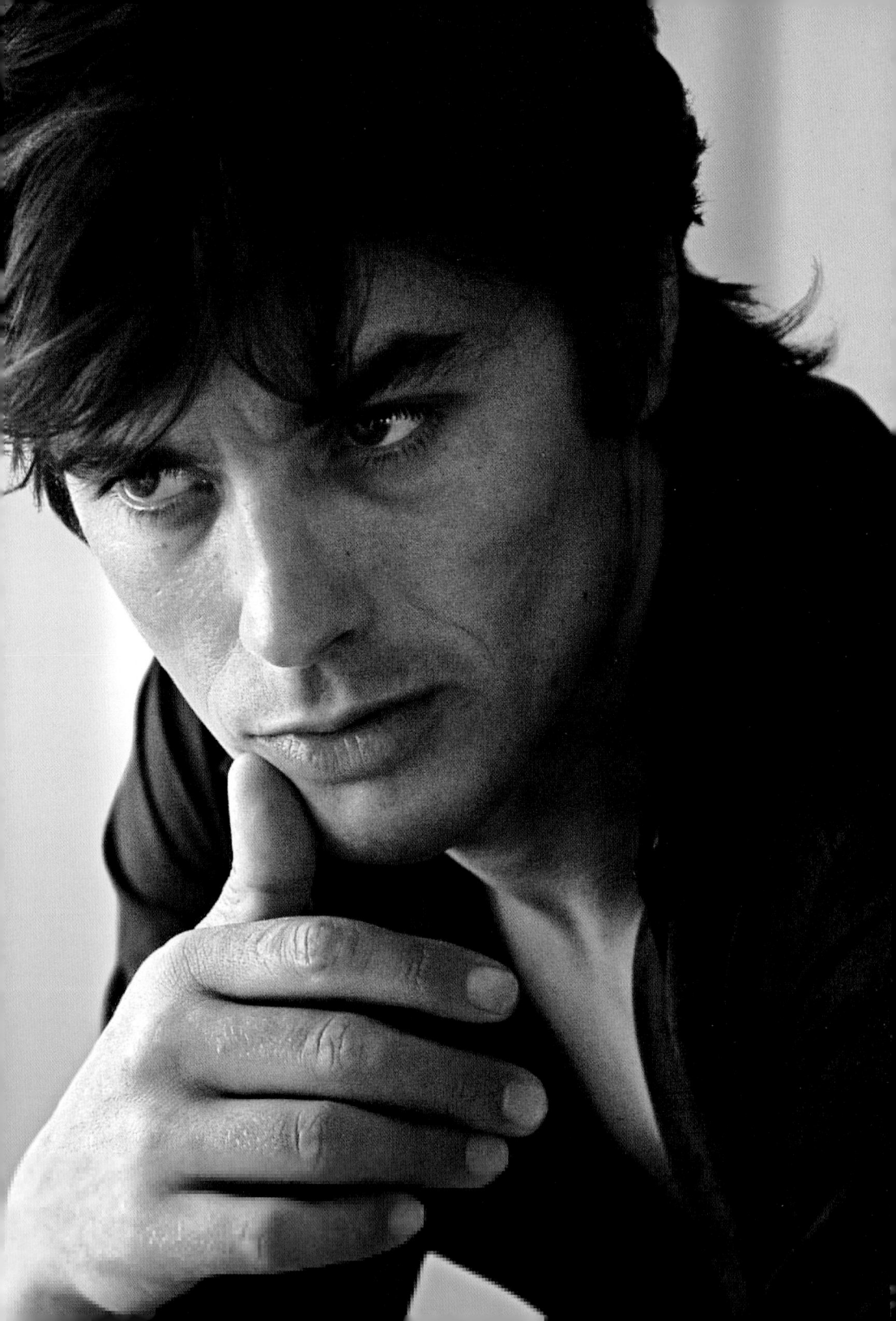

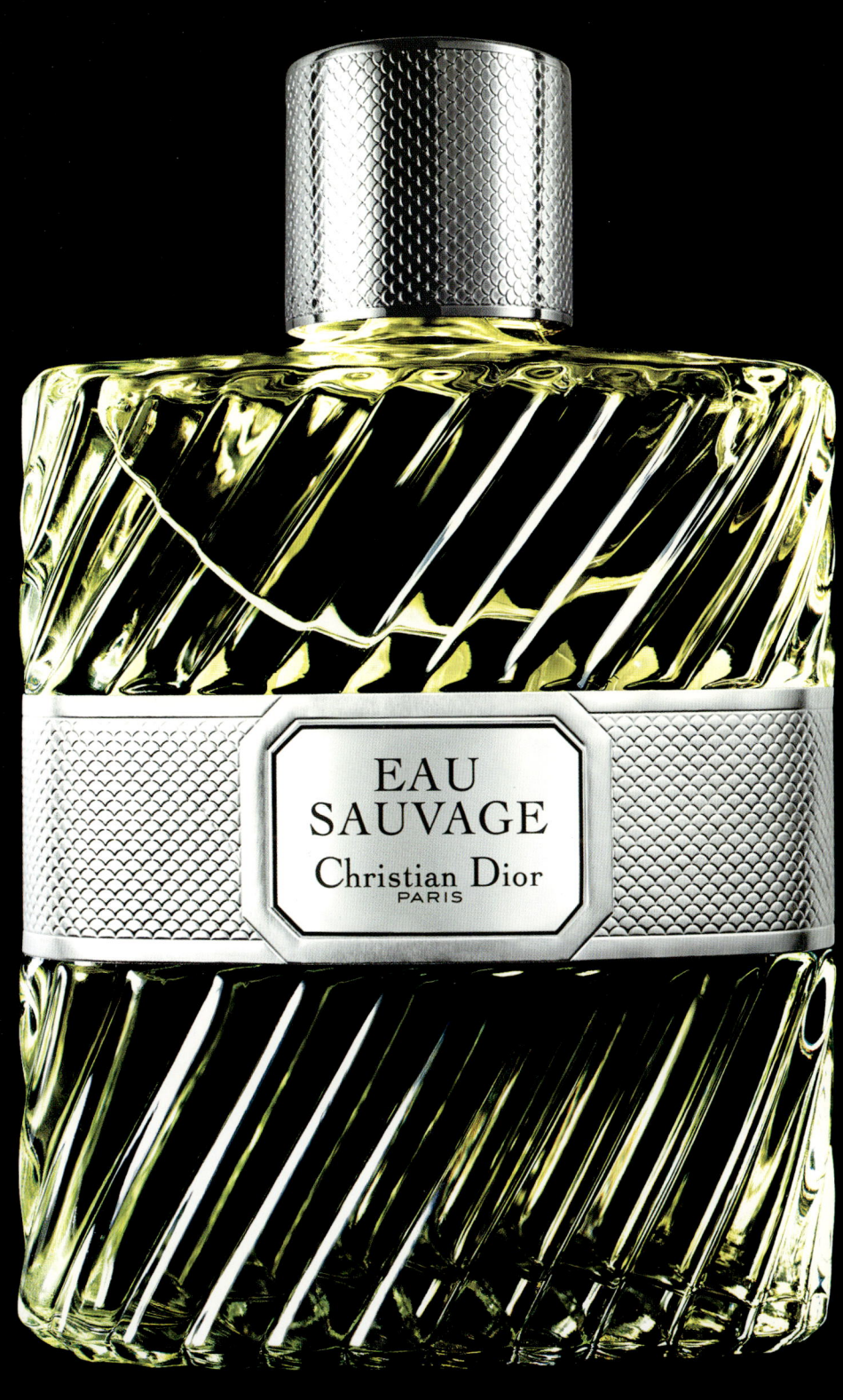

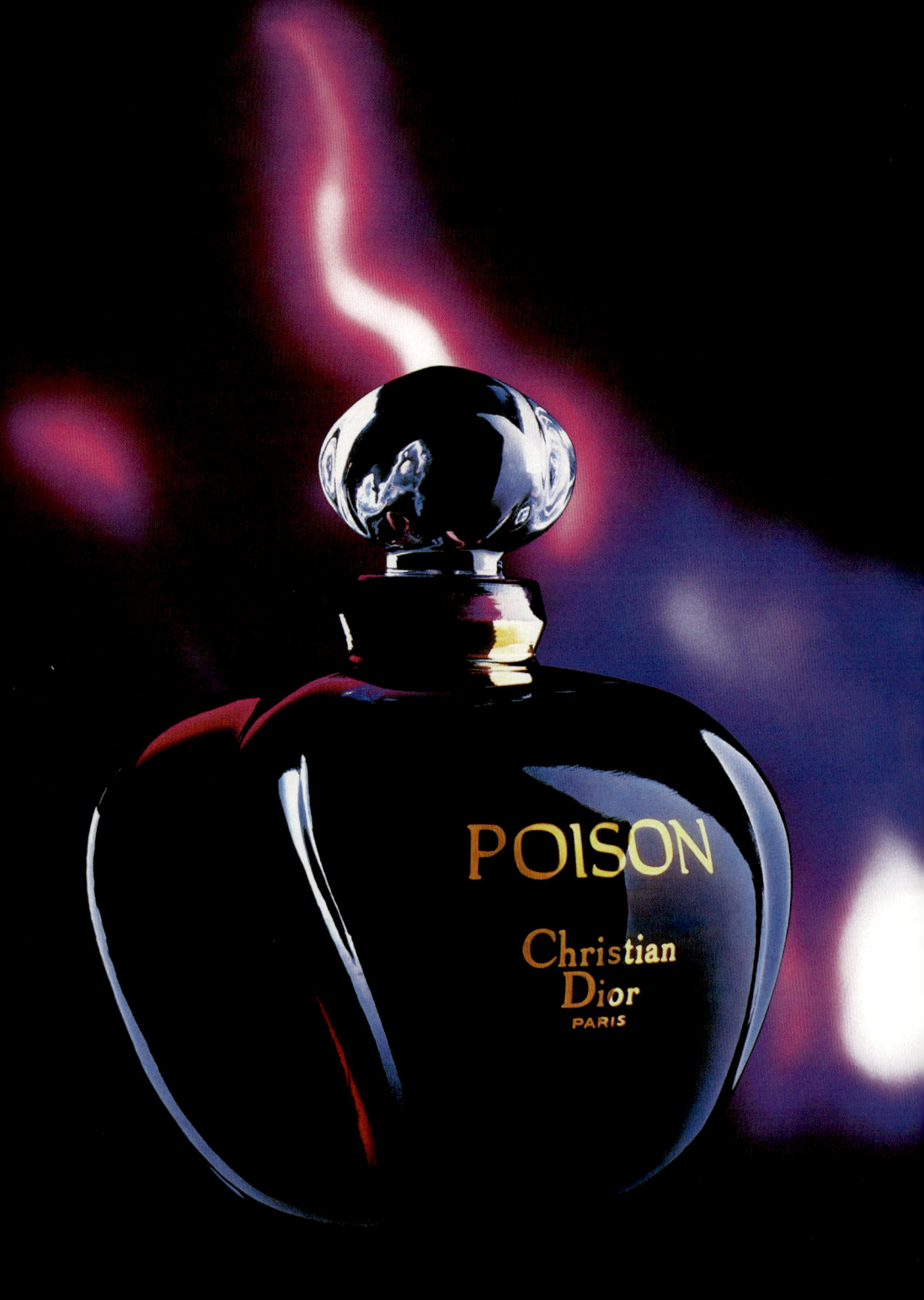

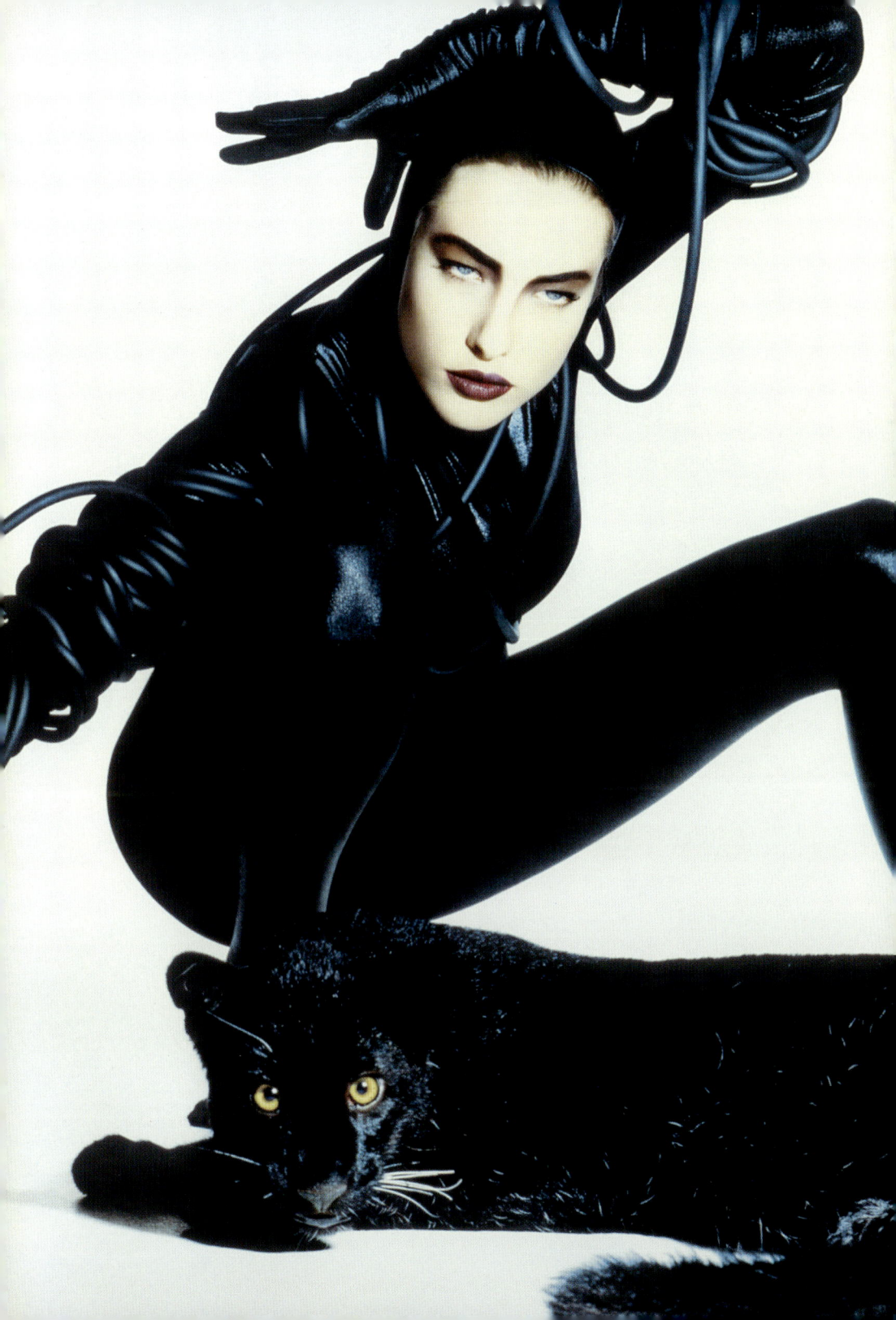

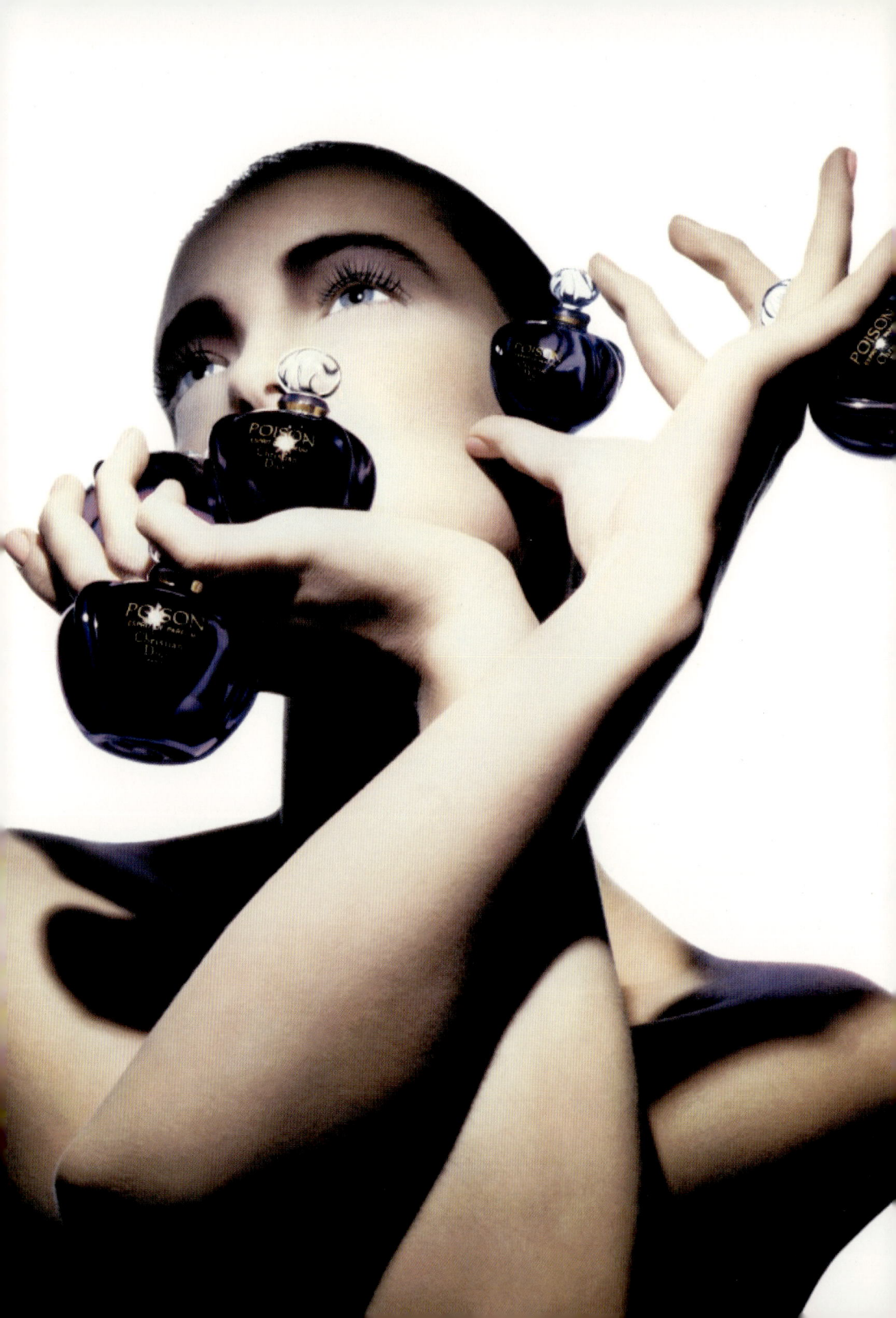

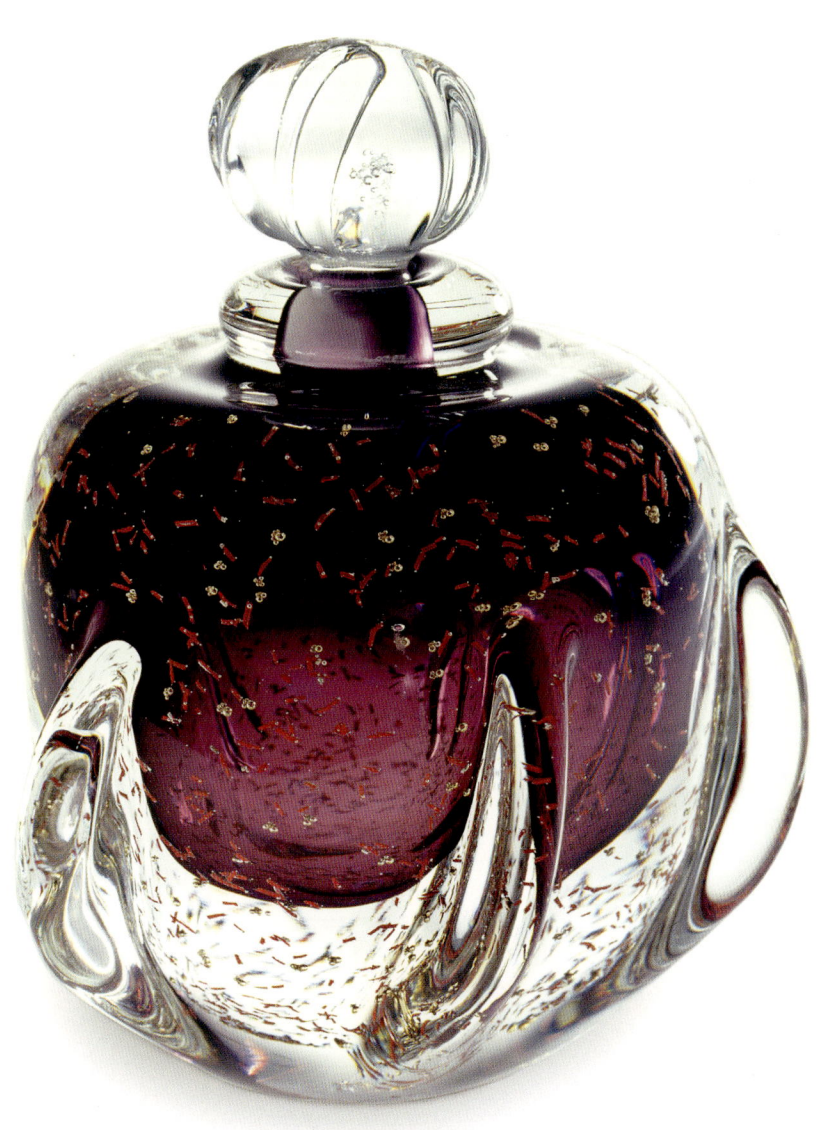

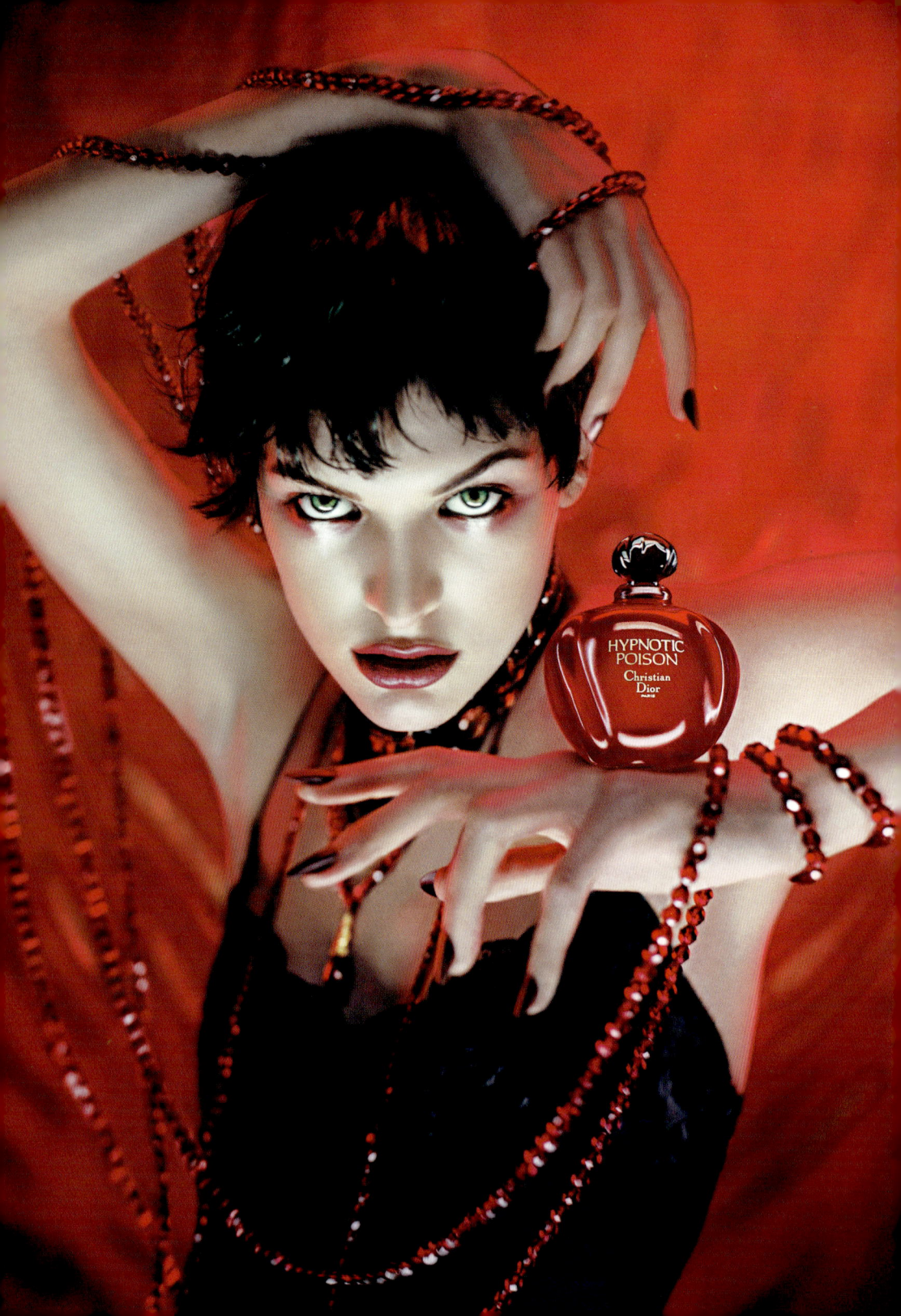

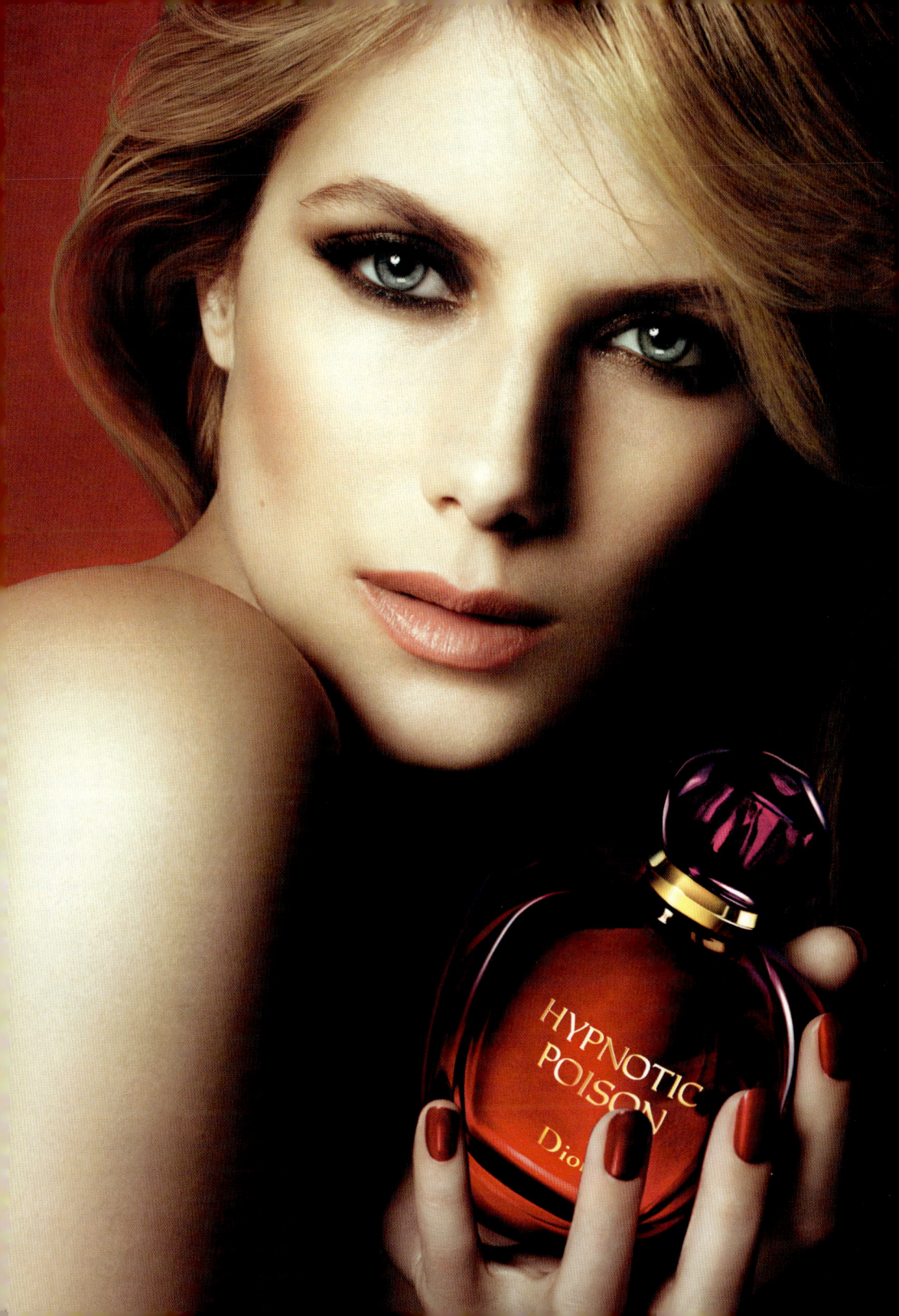

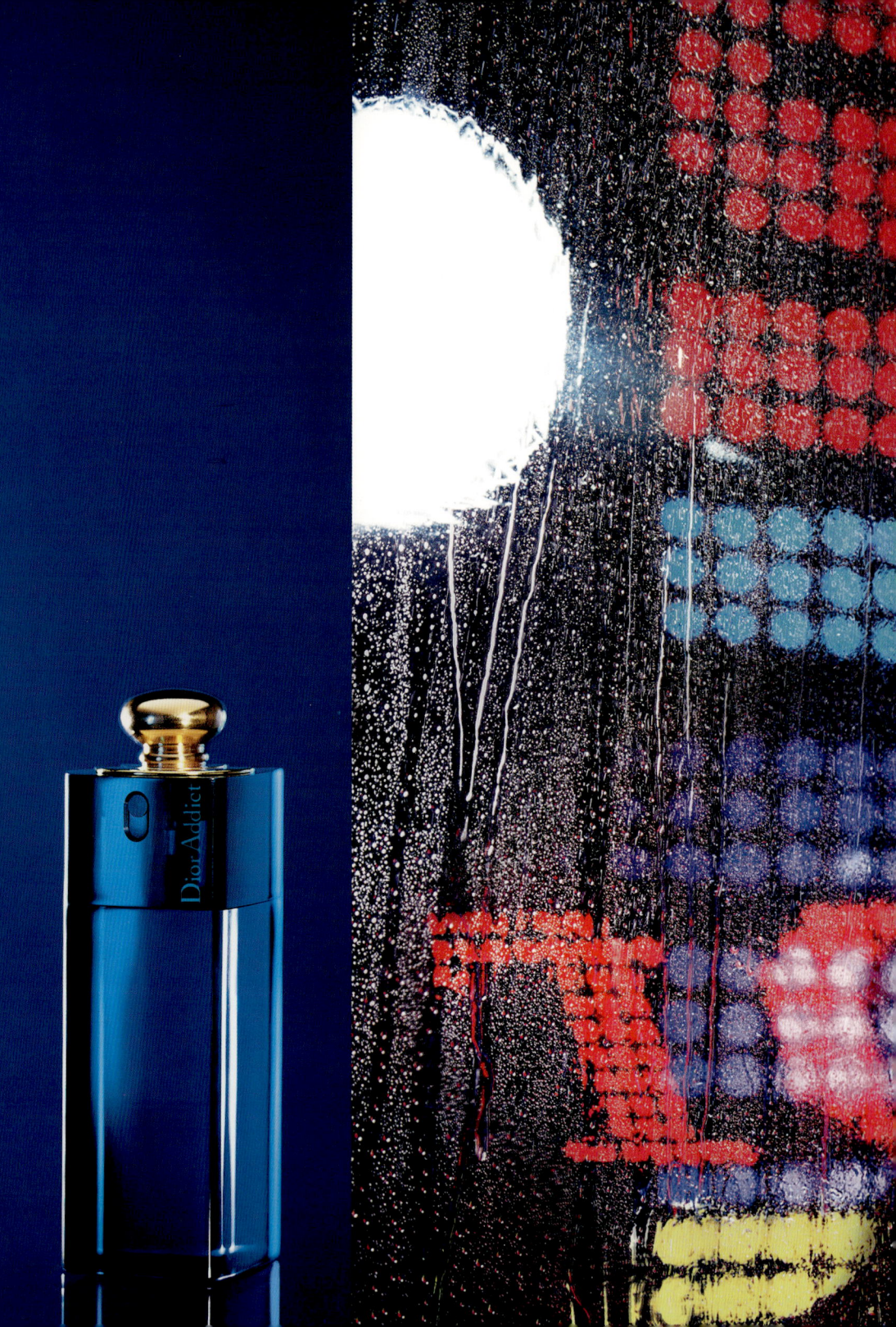

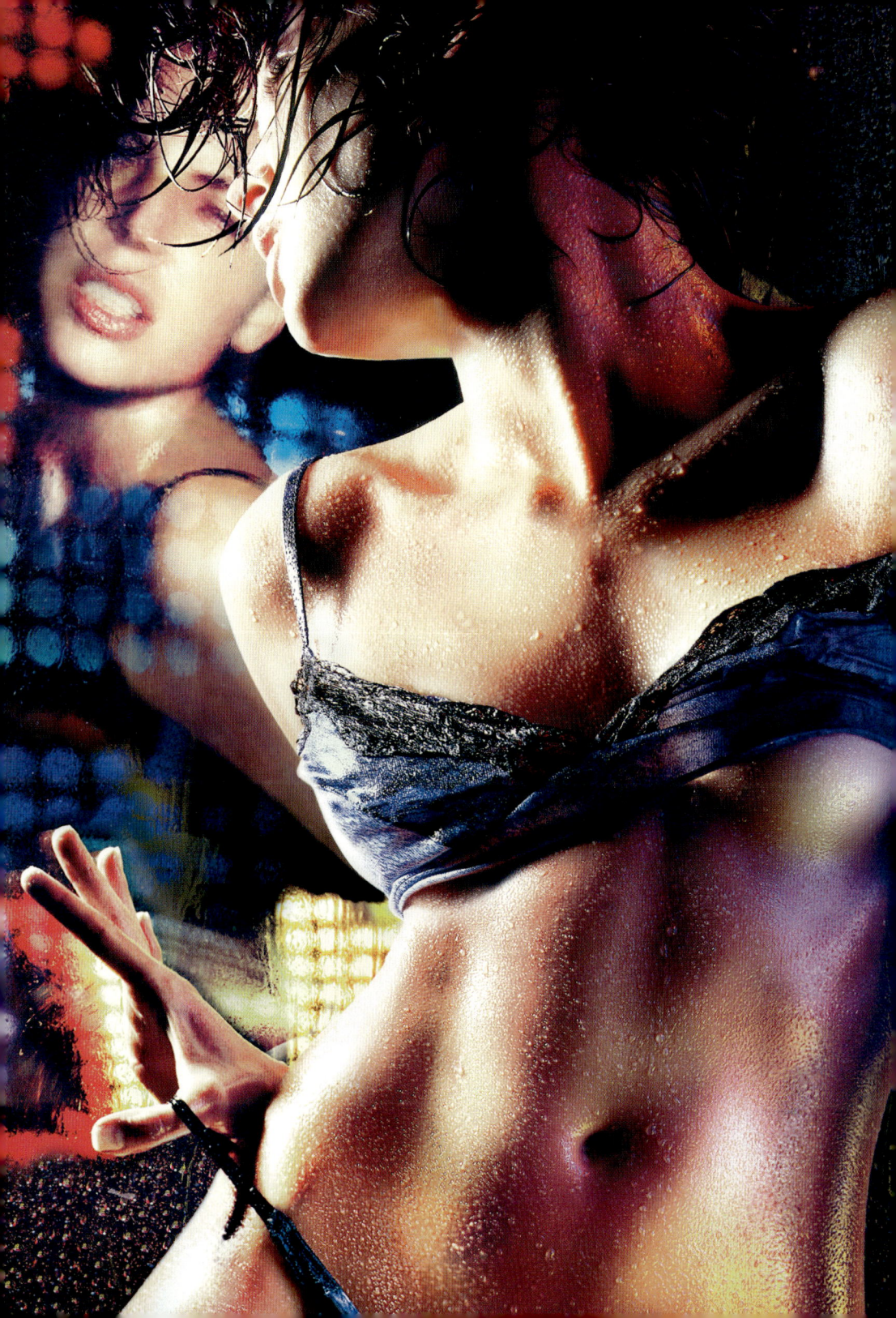

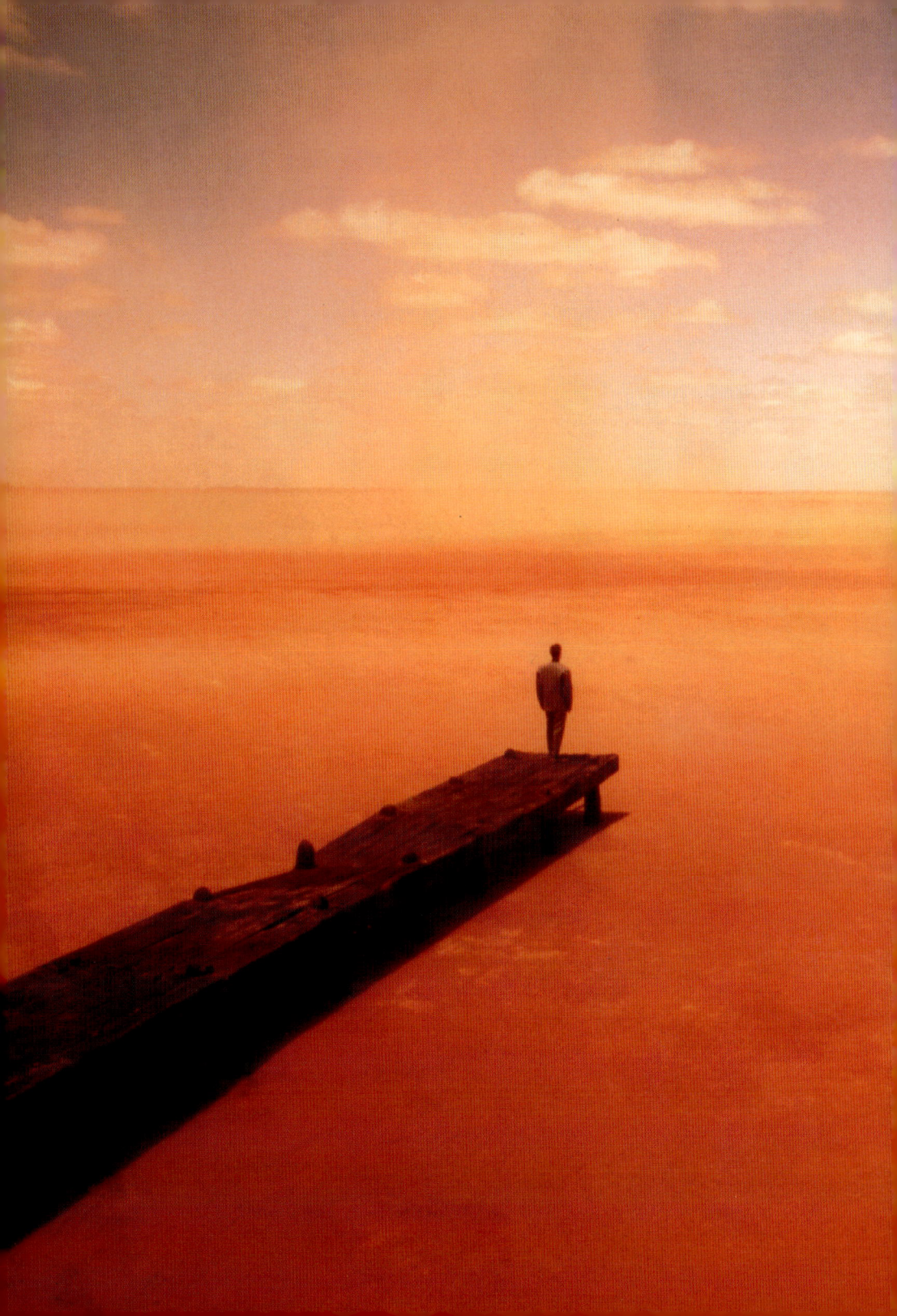

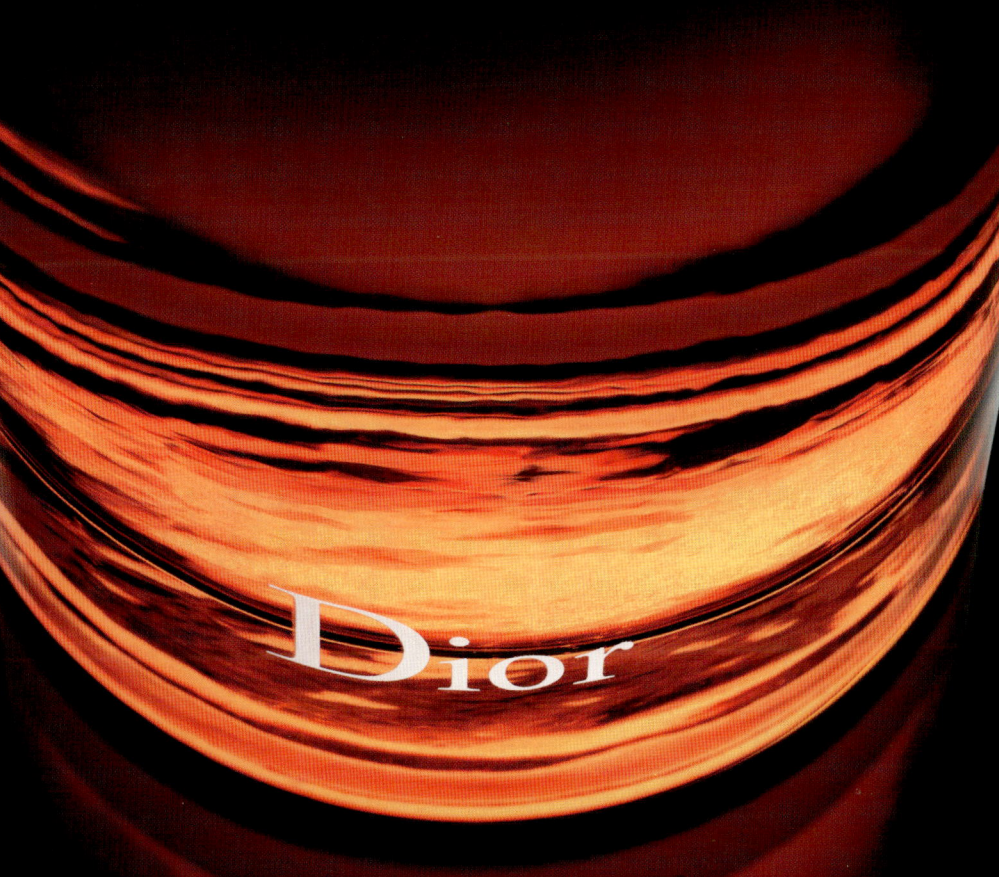

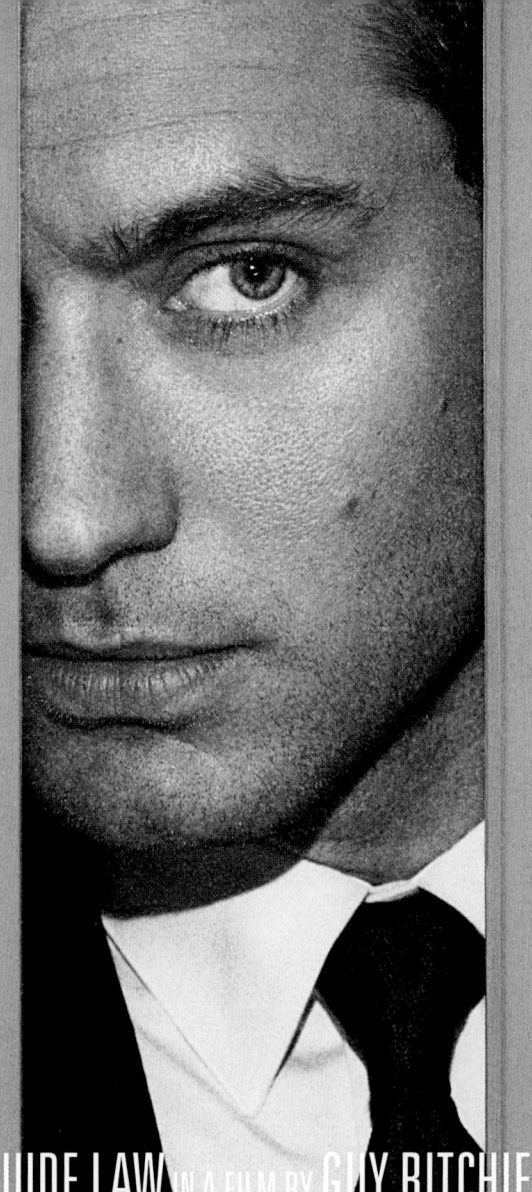

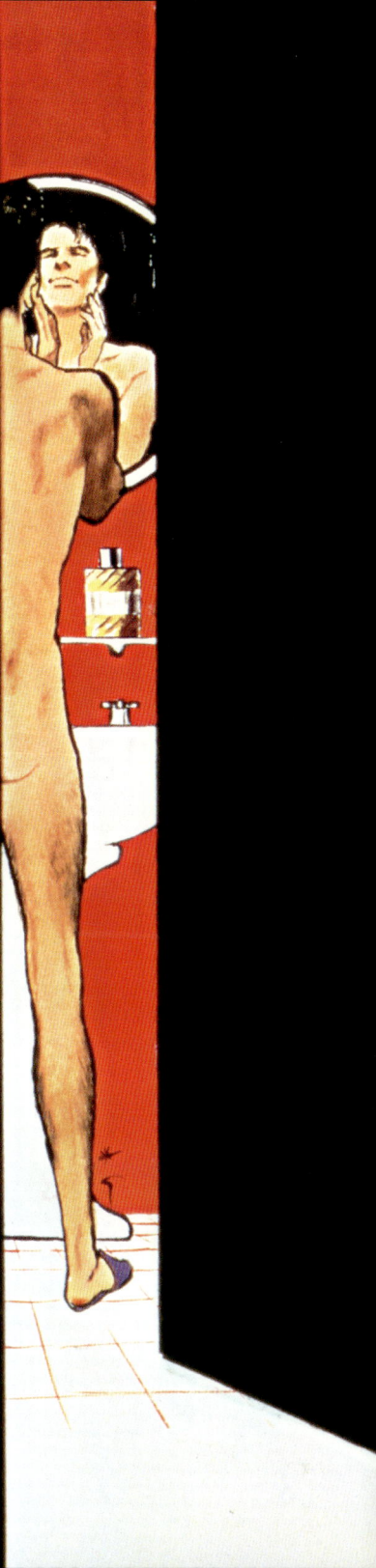

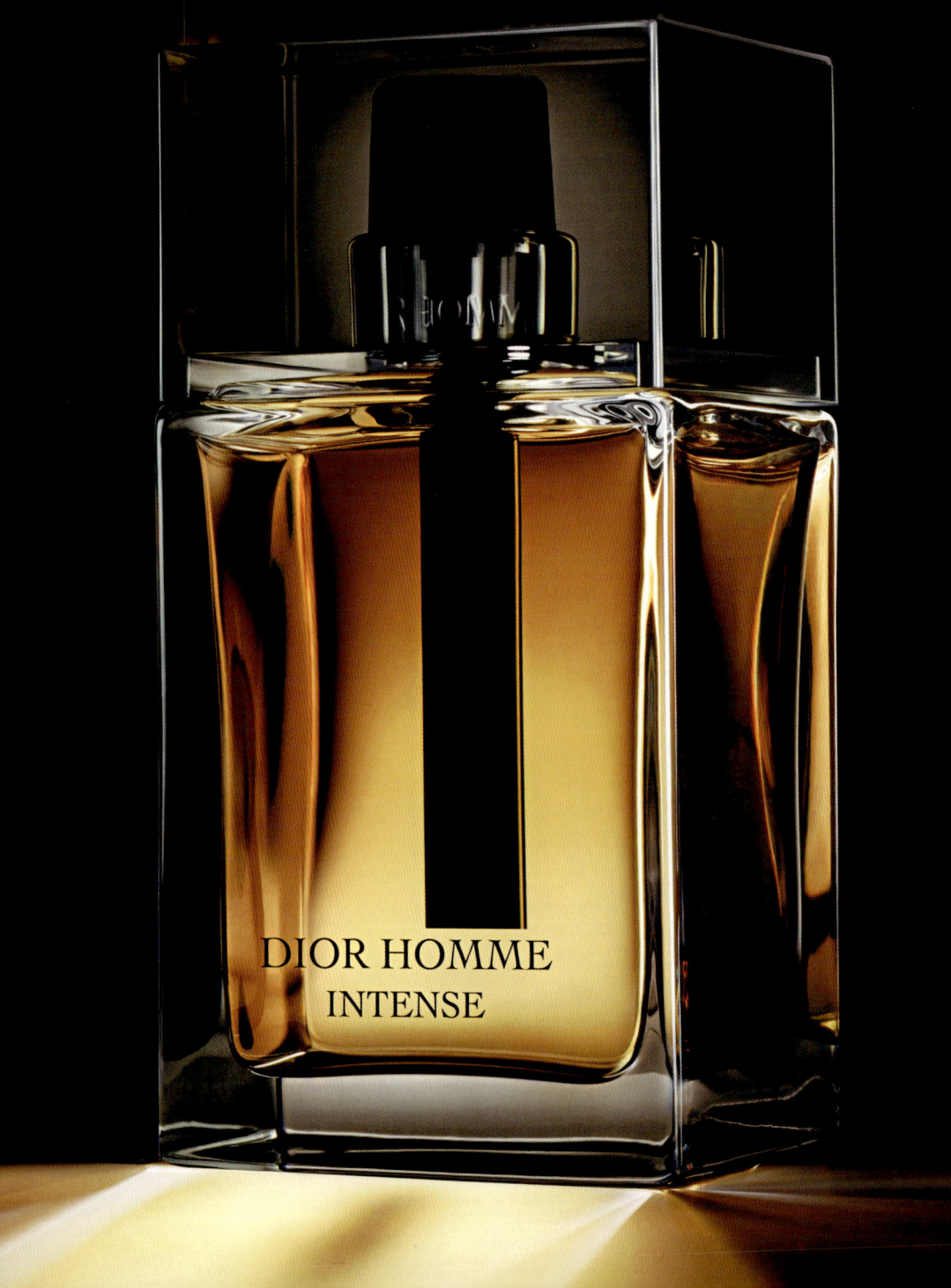

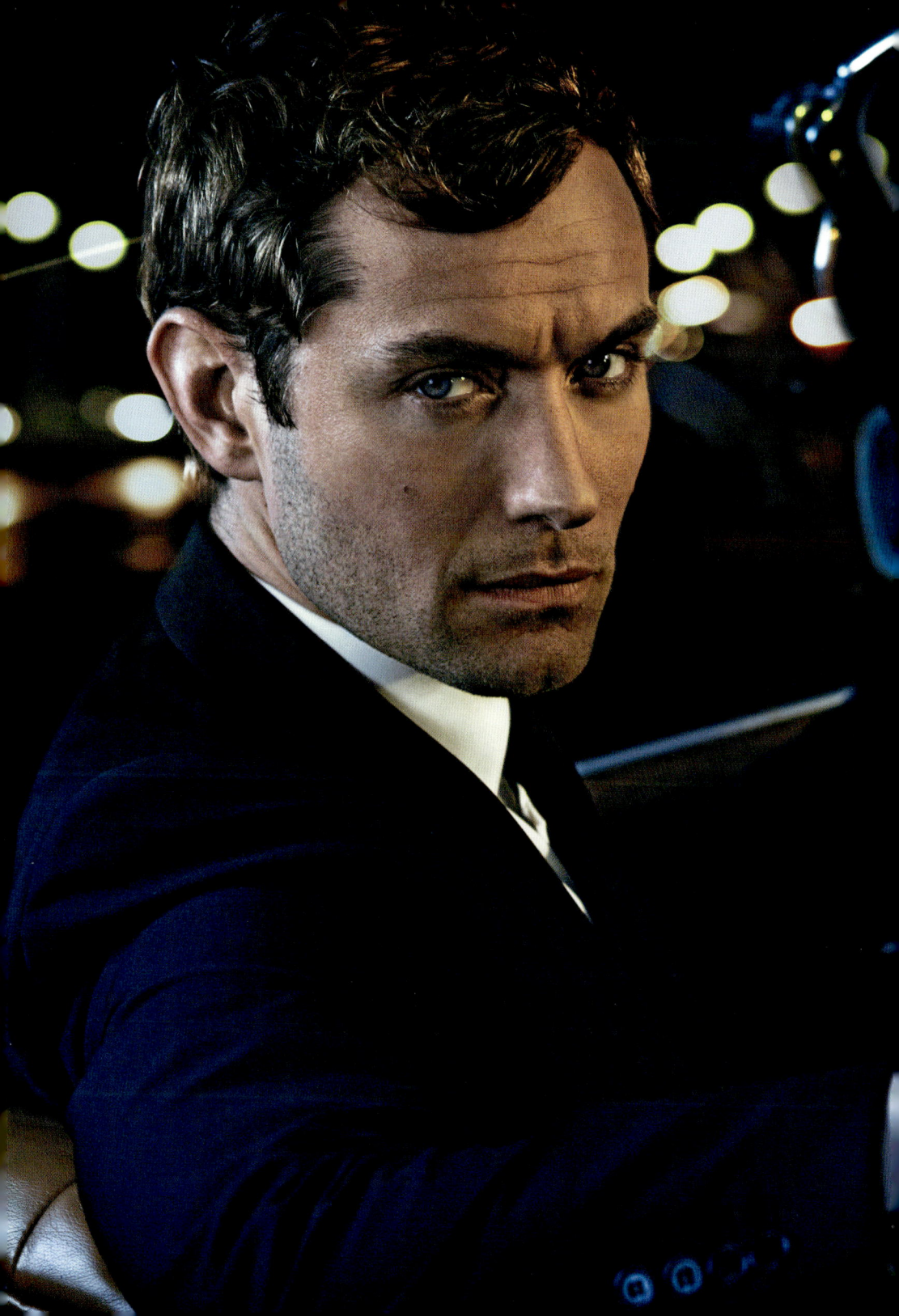

Notes

1. Christian Dior, interviewed circa 1950.
2. In order to be profitable, the perfume's life span must far exceed the seasonal nature of fashion.
3. Christian Dior wanted the most beautiful ingredients for his perfumes, the most noble raw materials of the highest quality. Today the House of Dior still uses flowers harvested exclusively for it, notably those from the Domaine de Manon in Grasse for jasmine and rose of May.
4. Edmond Roudnitska. Curriculum Vitae. In *Une Vie au service du parfum*, Thérèse Vian Éditions.
5. *Sous le signe du parfum: Edmond Roudnitska, Compositeur-Parfumeur*. Jocelyn and Jean-Paul Le Maquet. Marie-Christine Grasse. Jean-Claude Ellena. Éditions de l'Albaron, 1991.
6. Ever since Jicky, by Guerlain, in 1889—the first perfume to mix synthetic ingredients with natural essences—fragrant chemical compounds have revolutionized perfumery. Today they are present in every creation, and the perfume creator's possibilities are severely limited without them. Some can be quite harsh or brutal, however, so throughout the first half of the twentieth century perfumers softened them by using a high proportion of vanilla, fruity, or sweet notes. It is known as sweet or candy perfumery (see Edmond Roudnitska).
7. Edmond Roudnitska. Curriculum Vitae. In *Une Vie au service du parfum*, Thérèse Vian Éditions.
8. Spring-Summer 1950.
9. A perfume trilogy created by the house perfumer-creator, François Demachy: Escale à Portofino in 2008, Escale à Pondichéry in 2009 and Escale aux Marquises in 2010.
10. Christian Dior, lecture given for the French Civilization course at the Sorbonne University in Paris on August 3, 1955.
11. Spring-Summer 1955. There were three other outfits named Rosée in Christian Dior's lifetime: Fall-Winter 1947, Spring-Summer 1956, and Spring-Summer 1957.
12. Spring-Summer 1954; Fall-Winter 1952.
13. Fall-Winter 1953.
14. Spring-Summer 1949; Fall-Winter 1950; Fall-Winter 1953 and 1957; Fall-Winter 1956.
15. Translator's note: In order of mention, the English flower names are: acacia, daisy, petunia, reseda, forget-me-not, lily, iris, poppy, dahlia, hydrangea, lupine, carnation, colza, buttercup, angelica, and scabious.
16. Spring-Summer 1953.
17. Spring-Summer 1952.
18. Spring-Summer 1951; Spring-Summer 1952; Spring-Summer 1953.
19. Spring-Summer 1948; Spring-Summer 1949; Fall-Winter 1947.
20. Spring-Summer 1949; Spring-Summer 1951.
21. Fall-Winter 1950 and 1952.
22. *Sous le signe du parfum: Edmond Roudnitska, Compositeur-Parfumeur*. Le Maquet et al.
23. Speech given in Monte Carlo by Maurice Roger, then president of Parfums Christian Dior, on June 17, 1985, for the launch of Poison.
24. In the 1980s, the world of perfumery entered a period of highly competitive transformation. To stand out, the launch of Poison enjoyed a huge budget for its day. Advertising campaign, commercial directed by Claude Chabrol, a grand ball held for the official launch at the Château Vaux-le-Vicomte in France—a global communications budget estimated at $40 million.
25. Speech by Maurice Roger in Monte Carlo.
26. Christian Dior, *Je suis couturier*. Interviewed by Alice Chavane and Elie Rabourdin. Éditions du Conquistador (1951, out of print).

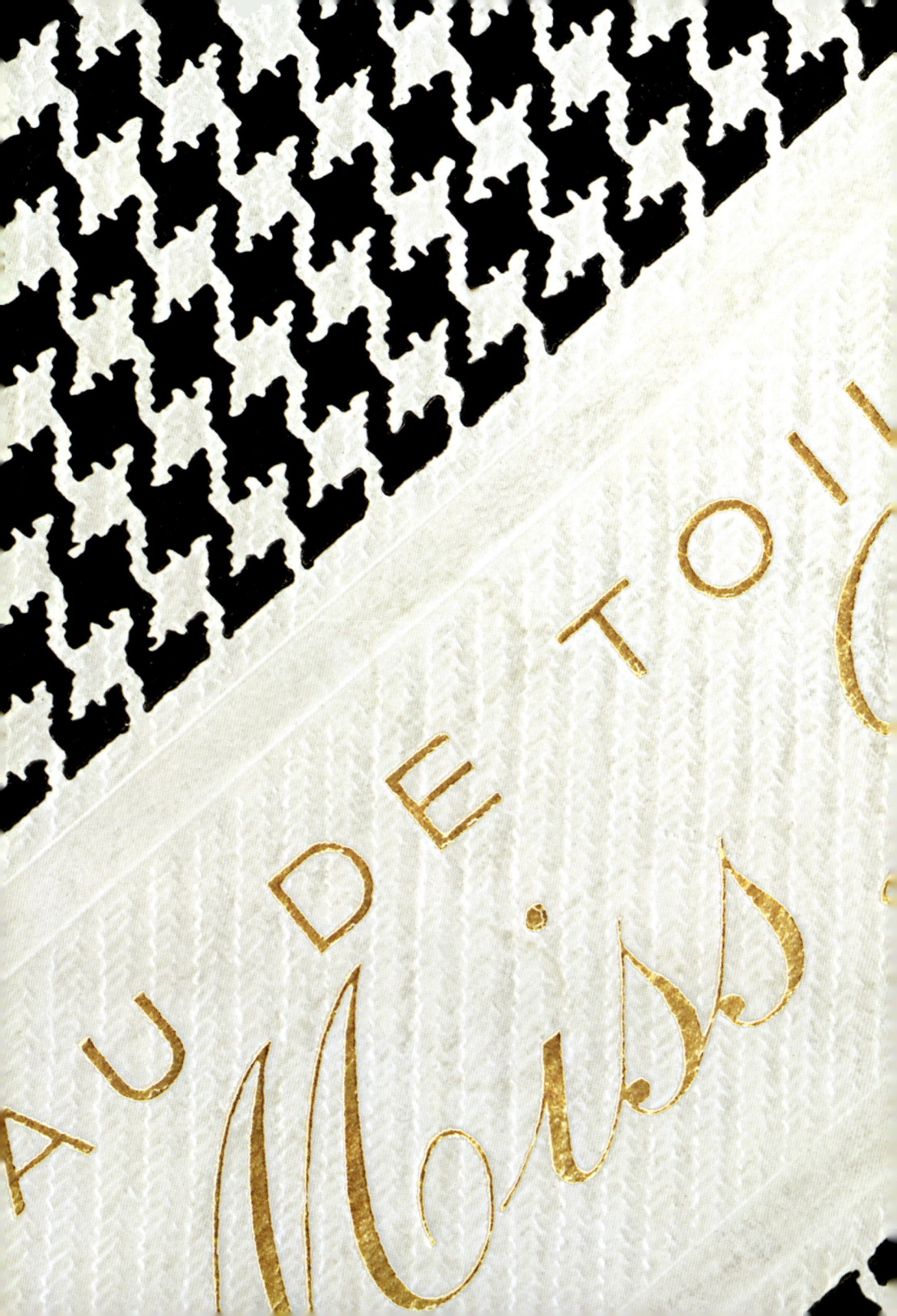

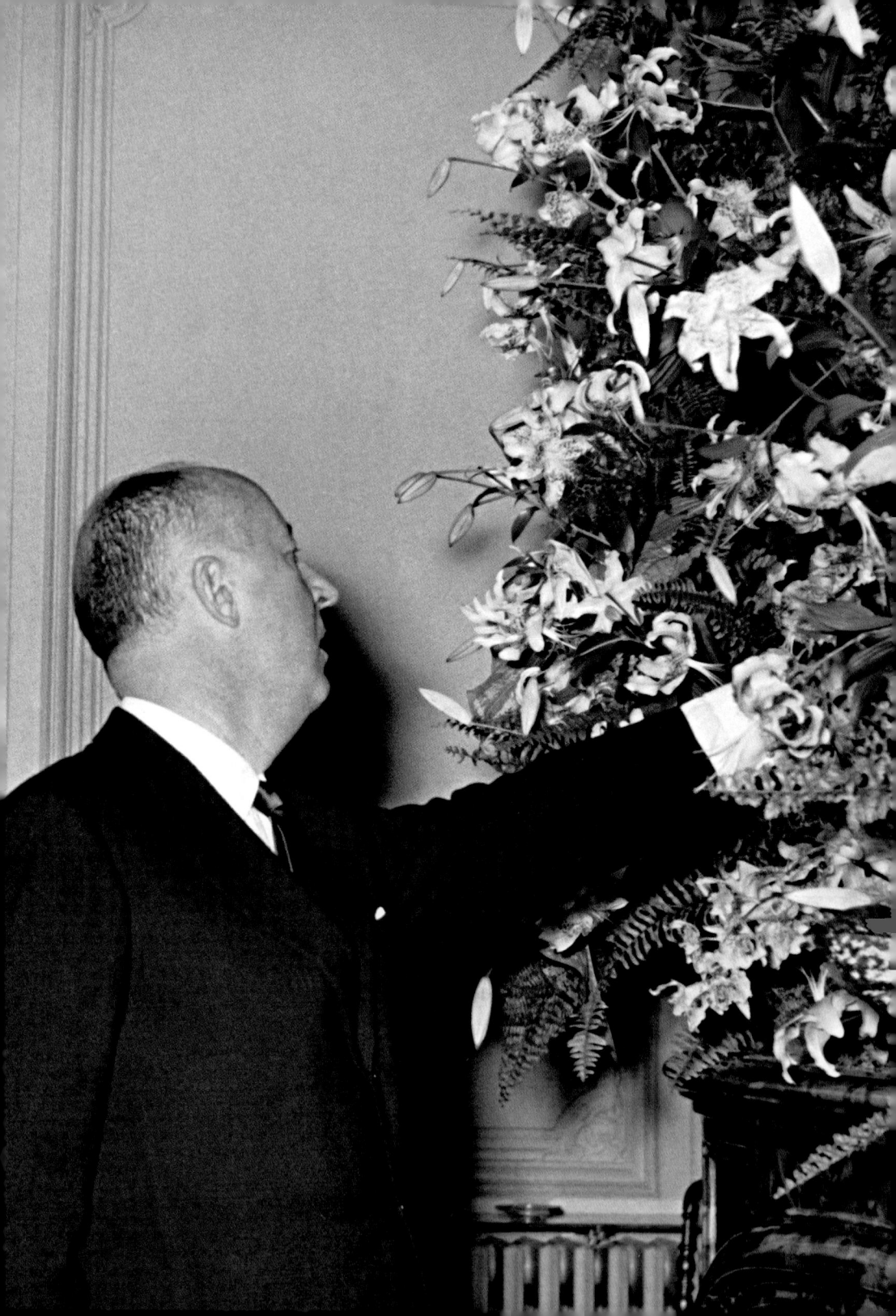

Chronology

1947:	Introduction of Miss Dior at the New Look couture show, February 12.
1949:	Launch of Diorama, the first perfume created by Edmond Roudnitska.
1955:	Launch of L'Eau Fraîche, the first unisex eau de cologne.
1956:	Launch of Diorissimo, Dior's good luck perfume.
1963:	Launch of Diorling.
1966:	Launch of L'Eau Sauvage for men with a complete line of products, a first in perfumery.
1972:	For the launch of Diorella, René Gruau draws the first Dior woman to wear pants in an advertisement.
1979:	Dioresscence was first introduced in 1973 as a bath line, then as a perfume.
1980:	Launch of Jules, the first sport fragrance by Christian Dior Perfumes.
1985:	Launch of Poison at the Vaux-le-Vicomte château, September 17.
1988:	Launch of Fahrenheit.
1998:	Launch of Hypnotic Poison.
1999:	Launch of J'adore.
2002:	Launch of Dior Addict.
2005:	Launch of Dior Homme.
2008:	Launch of Escale à Portofino.
2011:	La Collection Privée Christian Dior.

Christian Dior at 30 Avenue Montaigne, circa 1955. The couturier himself saw to the flower arrangements and encouraged his staff to spritz the salons with Dior perfumes. Photo © 2011 Association Willy Maywald/Artists Rights Society (ARS), New York/ADAGP, Paris

Dior
PERFUME

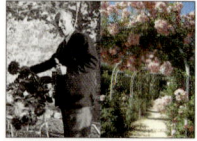
Christian Dior in his garden at Milly-la-Forêt, circa 1953. A great connoisseur of flowers and their fragrances, Dior designed the gardens at his houses at Milly-la-Forêt and Montauroux himself. Photo © André Ostier. **Flowers from the garden at villa Les Rhumbs in Granville, Dior's childhood home.** Christian Dior acquired a passion for roses very early in life, inspired by their colors, shapes, and delicate scent. Photo © 2008 Musée Christian Dior.

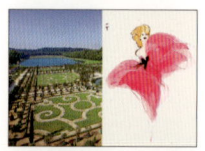
The gardens at Versailles Palace and the style of the court of the Sun King inspired Christian Dior's fragrance creations. Photo © Jose Fuste Raga/Corbis. **Illustration by René Gruau for Miss Dior, 1961.** From 1947, Gruau celebrated his friend Christian Dior's "flower women," and his illustrations expressed the intangibility of perfume. Photo © SARL René Gruau/www.renegruau.com.

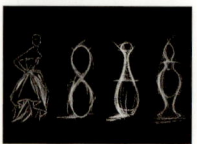
Christian Dior, couturier-perfumer. The evolution of the En Huit (Figure 8) line of 1947 to the amphora design of the original Miss Dior flacon to today's J'adore bottle. Christian Dior always believed that "Perfume is the finishing touch to a dress." Photo © 2010 Christian Dior Perfumes.

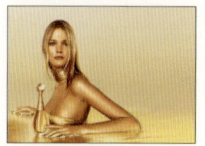
J'adore by Jean-Baptiste Mondino. The first campaign for J'adore, featuring model Carmen Kass, paid homage to the radiant power of absolute femininity. Photo: Jean-Baptiste Mondino © Christian Dior Perfumes.

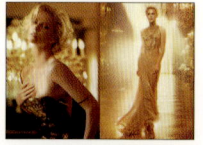
J'adore by Patrick Demarchelier. The face of Dior since 2004, Charlize Theron has revealed the personality of the fragrance through the lenses of the greatest photographers. Photo: Patrick Demarchelier © Christian Dior Perfumes. **J'adore by Jean-Jacques Annaud.** Filmed in the Hall of Mirrors at Versailles, this campaign for J'adore was an ode to femininity. Photo © 2011 Christian Dior Perfumes.

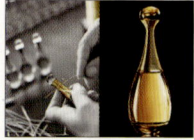
Applying the gold collar to the J'adore bottle. Faithful to its heritage of craftsmanship, Dior continues to refine the art of perfumery by releasing special editions, featuring touches such as frosted and hand-cut crystal, gilding, and engraving of the star motif, one of Christian Dior's lucky charms. Photo: Philippe Schlienger © 1999 Christian Dior Perfumes. **J'adore l'Absolue.** From eau de toilette to more concentrated versions, Dior uses the highest quality ingredients. Photo © 2010 Christian Dior Perfumes.

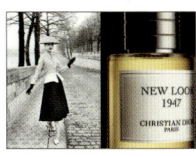
The Bar suit, 1947. The most famous ensemble from the first Christian Dior Haute Couture collection in February 1947, the Bar suit represented the new, more architectural standard of classic Parisian elegance. Photo © 2011 Association Willy Maywald/Artists Rights Society (ARS), New York/ADAGP, Paris. **New Look 1947**, one of the fragrances in La Collection Privée, which marries couture and perfumery traditions to produce modern expressions of the master's vision. Photo © 2011 Christian Dior Perfumes.

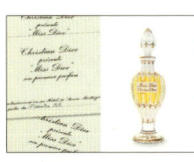
Invitation to the launch of Miss Dior, 1947. As with his Haute Couture collections, Dior celebrated the launch of his first fragrance by inviting clients and journalists to 30 Avenue Montaigne. With Miss Dior, he wanted to create "a perfume with the fragrance of love." Photo © Christian Dior Perfumes. **The original Baccarat crystal Miss Dior amphora bottle, 1951**, with opalescent crystal overlaid on clear crystal, the subtle play of materials expressing the refinement of Dior Haute Couture. Photo: Philippe Schlienger © Christian Dior Perfumes.

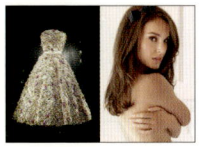
Miss Dior dress from the Spring-Summer 1949 Haute Couture collection. The allover floral embroidery of the Miss Dior cocktail dress calls to mind the flowers used in the perfume, the dress becoming an expression of the fragrance. Photo © Laziz Hamani. **Natalie Portman.** The face of Miss Dior, Natalie Portman embodies the romantic and saucy young Dior woman from yesterday to today. Photo: Tim Walker © 2010 Christian Dior Perfumes.

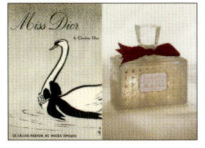
Miss Dior by René Gruau, 1949. Christian Dior and Gruau shared a love of classicism. The pearl-white swan, symbol of youth in the 18th century, was used by Gruau for the first Miss Dior advertisement. Photo © SARL René Gruau/www.renegruau.com. **Miss Dior bottle, 1950.** After the amphora, Christian Dior designed a more architectural version for Miss Dior, incorporating the bow and houndstooth pattern. Photo © Christian Dior Perfumes.

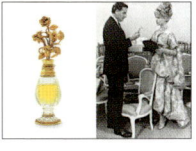
The original Baccarat crystal flacon for Diorissimo, designed by Christian Dior, 1956. This edition was topped with a floral bouquet stopper in fine gold, representing the flowers in the perfume. Photo © Christian Dior Perfumes. **Brigitte Bardot receiving Diorissimo at 30 Avenue Montaigne, 1960.** Undeniable icon of the 1960s, Brigitte Bardot was invited to discover the single-floral Diorissimo fragrance by Edmond Roudnitska, an expression of lily of the valley, Christian Dior's favorite flower. Photo © Christian Dior Perfumes.

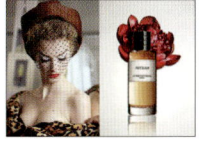
Mitzah Bricard. Leopard-print ensemble from the Fall-Winter 2009 Haute Couture collection, in homage to Mitzah Bricard, Christian Dior's muse and ally; he thought of her as the ambassador of refinement. Photo: Thibaut de Saint-Chamas. **Mitzah, one of the fragrances in La Collection Privée.** In 2010, François Demachy created a sensual oriental perfume for Dior christened Mitzah, a fragrance recalling the feline and spiritual femininity of Mitzah Bricard. Photo © Laziz Hamani.

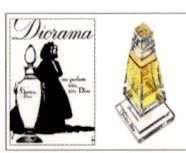

Diorama by René Gruau, 1961. A Venetian Carnival disguise was chosen to represent Diorama. René Gruau paid homage to the grand society balls so dear to Christian Dior in the 1950s. Photo © SARL René Gruau/www.renegruau.com. **Diorama Obelisk flacon, 1955.** Created in clear Baccarat crystal, this limited edition recalls the obelisk of the Place de la Concorde and Christian Dior's love of Paris. Photo: Philippe Schlienger © Christian Dior Perfumes.

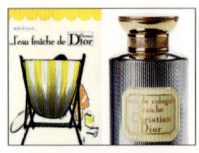

Eau Fraîche by René Gruau, 1955. The illustrator chose a sporty ambience for the first cologne by Christian Dior Perfumes. Photo © SARL René Gruau/www.renegruau.com. **Eau de Cologne Fraîche, 1955.** Early on, Christian Dior launched travel editions for his international clientele. Flacons in silvertone metal were designed for Eau Fraîche to better preserve the fragrance. Photo: Philippe Schlienger © Christian Dior Perfumes.

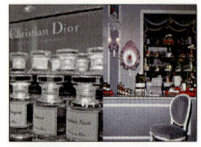

Fine ingredients. The same way the best fabrics are chosen for Haute Couture, the fragrance components are selected according to the highest standards of quality and provenance. Photo © 2010 Christian Dior Perfumes. **The 18th century.** In this 1955 photograph of the Christian Dior Parfums boutique, the grand decorative motifs of the 18th century can be seen: Trianon gray, the Fontange bow, and sunray pleats all serve to showcase the Dior fragrances and cosmetics. Photo © Christian Dior Perfumes.

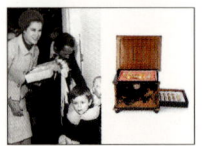

Princess Grace of Monaco at the opening of the Baby Dior boutique in 1967. The first collection designed for children, Baby Dior offered a range of products, including an eau de cologne. Photo: Courtesy Christian Dior Archives. **Chest of Christian Dior Perfumes offered to Princess Grace of Monaco in 1961.** This 19th-century lacquered box contained a luxury edition of Diorissimo perfume and an assortment of 14 Dior lipsticks. Photo © Philippe Schlienger.

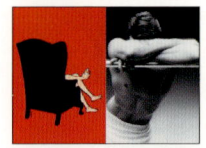

Eau Sauvage by Gruau, 1978. René Gruau could depict everyday situations with humor and a wink of impertinence. The nude gentleman here holds a flacon of Eau Sauvage in place of a glass of whiskey. Photo © SARL René Gruau/www.renegruau.com. **Eau Sauvage by Dominique Issermann.** This emblematic visual from 1987 is the first photograph for an Eau Sauvage campaign after the ones illustrated by Gruau. "The man at the barre" offered a new virile and mysterious image for Eau Sauvage. Photo © Dominique Issermann.

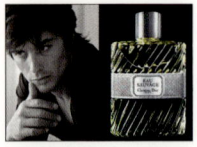

Eau Sauvage by Jean-Marie Périer, 1966. Classic and timeless, Eau Sauvage is the fragrance of great modern legends, such as Alain Delon, who represents the eternal masculine. Photo © Jean-Marie Périer. **Eau Sauvage flacon, 1966.** This bottle, created by Pierre Carnin, is a modern blend of feminine and masculine design styles. Photo © Christian Dior Perfumes.

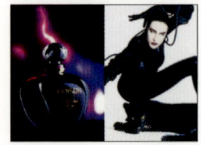

Poison by Tyen, 1985. Thanks to an extensive global campaign by Tyen and Claude Chabrol, Poison became a worldwide phenomenon that led to new versions such as Hypnotic Poison in 1998 and Pure Poison in 2006. Photos: Tyen © Christian Dior Perfumes.

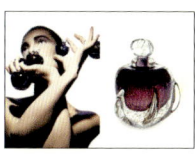

Poison by Tyen. In 1985, Poison wrote a new page in the history of Christian Dior, becoming the first in a new generation of perfumes inspired by an evocative name and the extreme possibilities of the world of fragrance. Photo: Tyen © Christian Dior Perfumes. **Poison bottle, 1985.** The flacon's form calls to mind a fruit or a volcano, two strong ideas embodied in the power of the perfume's oriental essences. Photo © Christian Dior Perfumes.

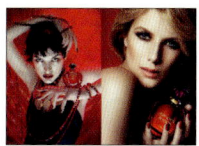

Milla Jovovich for Hypnotic Poison, 1998. Directed by Jean-Baptiste Mondino, the advertisement video for Hypnotic Poison featured a fascinating and possibly even dangerous woman, the ideal role for Milla Jovovich, who was first showcased by Luc Besson in 1997 in *The Fifth Element*. Photo © Jean-Baptiste Mondino. **Mélanie Laurent for Hypnotic Poison, 2011.** Photo © Christian Dior Perfumes.

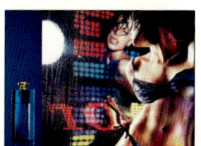

Dior Addict flacon, 2002. Photo © Christian Dior Perfumes. **Dior Addict by Nick Knight, 2002.** Dior Addict explores an unbridled sexiness, magnificently illustrated by the extreme visuals of Nick Knight. The use of avant-garde fashion photography is an electrifying step forward in the story of Christian Dior Perfumes. Photo © Nick Knight.

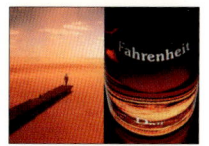

Fahrenheit by Ridley Scott. Upon its launch in 1988, Fahrenheit was a terrific success. The rich fragrance conjures images of wide-open spaces. Photo: Knut Bry © Christian Dior Perfumes. **The Fahrenheit bottle** is innovative, with its gradated sunset hues and profile reminiscent of a lighthouse. Photo: Laziz Hamani © 2010 Christian Dior Perfumes.

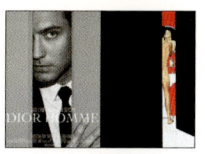

Still from an advertising video directed by Guy Ritchie for the Dior Homme campaign starring Jude Law, 2011. Photo: Peter Lindbergh © Christian Dior Perfumes. **René Gruau for Eau Sauvage, 1978.** Gruau helped define the image of modern masculinity by showing a man in the intimacy of the bathroom, an audaciously original setting. Photo © SARL René Gruau/www.renegruau.com.

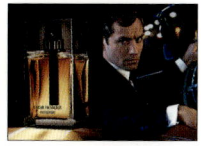

Dior Homme Intense, created in 2005. Dior Homme represents a strong and timeless masculinity, embodied by Jude Law since 2008. Photos © 2011 Christian Dior Perfumes.

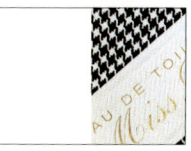

The Miss Dior packaging, 1950. Since 1947, Christian Dior applied his Haute Couture motifs to his perfume creations, like the houndstooth pattern, calligraphic script, and variations on the name "Dior," embodying the universe he created at 30 Avenue Montaigne and disseminating it around the world. Photo © Christian Dior Perfumes.

Acknowledgments

The publisher wishes to thank the Maison Dior for its help in the publication of this book.

Thanks also to: Denise Raab Jacobs; Thomas Michael Gunther, André Ostier; Sylvie Nissen, SARL René Gruau; Laziz Hamani; Alexandra Kadlec, Artists Rights Society; Anne Porto, Corbis.